Suffering
and Illness
Insights for
Caregivers

"Daedalus Mourning."

Suffering and Illness
Insights for Caregivers

Fay Carol Reed, PhD

 F. A. DAVIS COMPANY • Philadelphia

F. A. Davis Company
1915 Arch Street
Philadelphia, PA 19103
www.fadavis.com

Printed in the United States of America

Last digit indicates print number: 10 9 8 7 6 5 4 3 2 1

Acquisitions Editor: Lisa Biello
Developmental Editor: Melanie Freely
Production Editor: Nwakaego Fletcher-Perry
Cover Designer: Louis Forgione
Cover art: Landscape with the Fall of Icarus, by Pieter Bruegel the Elder
Chapter opening art: Daedalus Mourning, by Stuart Mark Feldman

As new scientific information becomes available through basic and clinical research, recommended treatments and drug therapies undergo changes. The author(s) and publisher have done everything possible to make this book accurate, up to date, and in accord with accepted standards at the time of publication. The author(s), editors, and publisher are not responsible for errors or omissions or for consequences from application of the book, and make no warranty, expressed or implied, in regard to the contents of the book. Any practice described in this book should be applied by the reader in accordance with professional standards of care used in regard to the unique circumstances that may apply in each situation. The reader is advised always to check product information (package inserts) for changes and new information regarding dose and contraindications before administering any drug. Caution is especially urged when using new or infrequently ordered drugs.

Library of Congress Cataloging-in-Publication Data

Reed, Fay Carol, 1934–
   Suffering and illness : insights for caregivers / Fay Carol Reed.
     p. ; cm
   Includes bibliographical references and index.
   ISBN 0-8036-1002-5 (papercover)
    1. Caregivers. 2. Suffering. 3. Sick—Psychology. 4. Stress (Psychology) I. Title.
   [DNLM: 1. Disease—psychology. 2. Stress, Psychological—prevention & control. WM 172 R323s 2003]
   R727.47 .R445 2003
   616'.001'9—dc21

2002067444

Preface

It may be foolhardy to attempt to write about suffering, for ultimately, it is experienced by a unique individual within a specific context and at a particular moment in time. Still, it is within our power as health-care professionals* to cause, to prevent, or to relieve suffering as well as to accompany patients† as they bear their unwelcome burden. Understanding how patients respond to illnesses that enfold suffering is an integral companion to the duty of curing disease and enhancing health. Although attention to suffering was once inherent in patient care, it is too often neglected in modern health-care practice and scholarship.

This work is intended to sharpen the reader's awareness and understanding of suffering and to furnish guidelines for caring for those who suffer. It is directed primarily to practicing clinicians and to students studying to become health-care professionals. It may also be valuable to those who wish to reflect on the suffering in their own lives or in the lives of others.

Part One examines the nature of suffering, how it is expressed, and what its significance may be, for without understanding how a particular patient suffers, relief may be difficult.

---

*The indefinite terms "health-care professional" and "clinician" are employed in order to be inclusive, although each profession offers particular competencies and specialized caring to sufferers.

†The word "patient" is used throughout this book, rather than contemporary labels such as consumer, guest, or client because it is unique to health care and because its very derivation comes from the Latin *patiens/ pati,* which means to suffer. (Simpson, J., & Weiner, E. (Eds.). (1989). *The Oxford English Dictionary.* Oxford, England: Claredon Press.)

Part Two builds upon this foundation, addressing how sufferers may be cared for. It focuses on patients' cognitive and experiential world and on the impact clinicians may have upon that world.

Efforts have been made to ground this book in the experience of real people in distress by drawing upon the author's own clinical experience and that of students and colleagues, as well as by including perspectives of suffering and related phenomena recorded in the literature of patient care and of related disciplines. Because attention to suffering *per se* is limited in health-care literature, writings from the humanities, which often transcend time and culture and serve as a repository of human experience, were also examined and incorporated. Brief excerpts from literature, including religious literature, are included because they capture the essence of suffering that has endured and been recorded from the classical period to modern times.

This work has recognizable limitations. It does not claim to capture all dimensions of suffering or the unique characteristics of acute suffering associated with specific diseases, disabilities, or conditions. Rather, this book focuses on the care of suffering adults who have experienced a physical illness or disability. The content assumes that these persons possess normal cognitive and emotional functioning and can communicate a sense of their past, present, and future. While it is recognized that patients have families and other significant relationships, are attached to various communities, and are culturally diverse, attention to these relationships would add undesirable length and undue complexity to this particular work.

The content is probably most pertinent to the majority culture in the United States, but it has broader relevance since some of the insights are drawn from the literature of various historical periods, religious perspectives, and cultures. Because this book focuses on suffering as an entity, it does not specifically address topics such as end-of-life care, euthanasia, and spiritual or personal growth through illness and suffering.

The general purposes of this book are to sensitize the reader to the existence of suffering, to delineate its general nature, to make the analysis useful in clinical practice, and ultimately, to ease suffering. The specific goals are to:

1. Recapture the significance of suffering in patient care by:
   a) Describing the common characteristics of suffering
   b) Enhancing clinicians' ability to more fully perceive and encounter suffering

      c) Familiarizing health-care professionals with some of the ways in which patients find significance in suffering

2. Make the identified characteristics useful in preventing or alleviating suffering by:

      a) Analyzing empathy and compassion as the initiators of care for suffering patients

      b) Identifying selected circumstances wherein patients suffer needlessly

      c) Enabling clinicians to particularize suffering

      d) Challenging health-care professionals to consistently incorporate the care of suffering persons into their practices

While suffering is not solely the domain of health-care professionals, these clinicians must be accountable for perceiving and addressing the suffering that is enmeshed in illness. Those who are committed to caring cannot allow suffering to remain mysterious and unstudied, or even worse, denied or neglected. Understanding and alleviating suffering is a challenge that is equal in complexity to discovering and validating the theories and techniques of the clinical sciences. Suffering is not a problem to be solved or treated in the same manner as science-based problems. It makes a different kind of demand on the clinician, which is to encounter the hurt and to uphold and, where possible, to heal the human being who suffers.

FAY CAROL REED, PHD, RN

Acknowledgements

Writing this book was made possible by the library staffs at Ohio
Wesleyan University and at the University of Cincinnati College of
Nursing, Doris Haag, Director. This book was also made possible by
the unseen persons in countless other libraries who secured and
forwarded materials that were essential to the completion of the work.
Recognition is due also to: Melanie Freely, who supported the proposal
that became this book; and to Lisa Biello, Acquisitions Editor; and
Marilyn Kochman, Developmental Editor, for their helpful suggestions,
clarifications, and diligence, which were essential to publication.
Preparation of the manuscript is credited to Laurel George's computer
competence, patience, and tireless effort.

Special appreciation is due to Corinne Reed Wilson, MEd, for her
unstinting assistance in crafting the language of the book, and to Ülle
Lewes, PhD, who made numerous suggestions about content and
resources. Additionally, the reviewers listed on page xi were extremely
helpful. I incorporated many of their thoughtful and substantive
comments with gratitude.

Finally, Dr. Mildred Newcomb merits particular thanks for her
early and sustained interest in this project, for her insightful criticism,
and for writing the Afterword, which added an important perspective
to the book.

Reviewers

Janet Geare Allen, MSN, RN, PHN, CRNH
Hospice and Palliative Care Program
Kaiser Permanente
Downey, California

Reverend Joseph A. Bracken, SJ
Professor
Director, Brueggeman Center
Xavier University
Cincinnati, Ohio

Karen Cummins, RN, MSN, CRNP
Professor of Nursing
Department Chair
Community College of Allegheny County
Pittsburgh, Pennsylvania

Cindy Davis, BSN, MNSc
Advanced Practice Women's Surgical Services
Central Arkansas Veterans Healthcare System
Little Rock, Arkansas

Nancy Dentlinger, BS, MS
Assistant Director of Nursing
Redlands Community College
El Reno, Oklahoma

Dia Campbell-Detrixhe, BSN, MSN
Nurse Educator/Course Coordinator
Redlands Community College
El Reno, Oklahoma

John Collins Harvey, MD, PhD
Professor of Medicine Emeritus
Georgetown University Medical Center
Georgetown University
Washington, DC

Bette Ide, RN, MA, PhD
Associate Professor and Director of Rural Health
  Specialization
College of Nursing
University of North Dakota
Grand Forks, North Dakota

Carol Kenner, DNS, RNC, FAAN
Associate Dean for Academic Advancement
Professor, Clinical Nursing
University of Illinois at Chicago
Chicago, Illinois

Reverend Edna Mason, AB, DM
Former Chaplain, Dept. of Pastoral Care
Riverside Methodist Hospitals
Columbus, Ohio

Jeanine Young-Mason, EdD, RN, CS, FAAN
Professor and Director, Office for the Advancement
  of Nursing Education
School of Nursing
University of Massachusetts
Amherst, Massachusetts

Carol Meadows, MSSc, RNP, APN
College of Nursing
University of Arkanasa
Fayetteville, Arkansas

Carla Mueller, PhD(c), RN
Associate Professor
University of Saint Francis
Fort Wayne, Indiana

Brother Ignatius Perkins, OP, MSN, DNSc, MAEd, RN
Executive Vice President
The National Catholic Bioethics Centers
Washington, DC

Geralyn Spollett, MSN
Associate Professor
School of Nursing
Yale University
New Haven, Connecticut

Joni Thanavaro, RN, MSN
Assistant Professor of Nursing
St. Louis Community College of Meramec
St. Louis, Missouri

Rev. Emmanuel Twesigye, PhD
Professor
Department of Religion
Ohio Wesleyan University
Delaware, Ohio

Contents

PART ONE

Encountering Suffering

Chapter 1

Why Should Suffering Be Studied?

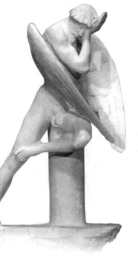

Musée des Beaux Arts
About suffering they were never wrong,
The Old Masters: how well they understood
Its human position; how it takes place
While someone else is eating or opening a window or just walking
   dully along; . . .
In Brueghel's Icarus, for instance: how everything turns away
Quite leisurely from the disaster; the ploughman may
Have heard the splash, the forsaken cry,
But for him it was not an important failure; the sun shone
As it had to on the white legs disappearing into the green
Water; and the expensive delicate ship that must have seen
Something amazing, a boy falling out of the sky,
Had somewhere to get to and sailed calmly on.

W. H. AUDEN (1945, P. 3)

In the Greek myth *Icarus,* Daedalus and his son Icarus escaped King
Minos' imprisonment by fashioning wings that they attached to
themselves with glue. Ignoring his father's pleas to fly a middle
course, the delighted Icarus flew too close to the sun, which melted
the glue. His wings came off, and Icarus fell tragically into the sea
(Hamilton, 1942, p. 193). In the landscape by Breughel (cover),
Icarus's fall is unnoticed.

   Like Icarus, those who bear suffering know that it is at best a
lonely and fear-filled affair, often unrecognized by others. Although
suffering is experienced by nearly everyone, those who endure it may
conceal it. When others do perceive a person's suffering, they may
turn away because of their unwillingness or inability to face the
misery of another person. Even health-care professionals, who should
be sensitive to suffering, sometimes withdraw from those who suffer

3

because they are unsure how to proceed or they fear making matters worse. Often they are overwhelmed by other responsibilities.

In 1878, when the Rev. S. Baring-Gould wrote, "Who does not know that suffering and sorrow surrounds him on every side?" (p. 4), his query was merely rhetorical. Today the question invites consideration of whether people in general and health-care professionals in particular are aware of the depths of misery of persons who are suffering. How strange it seems that suffering and its relief, which are central to the mission of health care, are mentioned so infrequently in many hospitals and within the health-care delivery system.

Although there is much talk in clinical conferences about treatment strategies, physical symptom management, and patient care outcomes, it would be quite remarkable to discover a case conference planned to address, "The Suffering of John T, Room 310." The successes of modern science convey the impression that suffering has been conquered, but sensitive observation in any health-care environment demonstrates that suffering is pervasively present.

Relief of Suffering Is Intentional

Alleviating suffering or being present with a sufferer requires courage, sensitivity, competence, and work. Often the medical diagnosis is minimally helpful in determining either the nature or the intensity of the suffering that a patient experiences, although knowledge of disease processes and skillfully applied treatments obviously can and do relieve much suffering. The very personnel, institutions, and agencies from which patients seek care, moreover, sometimes cause suffering, even when care is scientifically correct. Patients within the health-care system may suffer not only from pathology but also from feeling socially isolated, dependent, and undignified. Sometimes, too, they are forced to choose between equally unacceptable alternatives of treatment or illness management without adequate information or support in the decision making.

Neither can suffering be treated or "fixed" easily—if at all. It is not merely physical pain; a person's inner experience is embodied. Usually suffering is a condition more akin to a syndrome with multiple etiologies and varied presentations or symptoms than to a disease that may be described specifically and treated with precision. Suffering is most commonly manifested in the context of dying, pain, and sickness. Often it varies in source and intensity from day to day or even from hour to hour in a single patient, and for some patients, suffering may have no end. Although general characteristics of suffering can be detected, suffering remains a unique personal experience that only the sufferer is able to perceive yet may be unable to articulate fully. To date, research has not provided a tested normative model of suffering; in fact, limited research appears to be under way.

Evolution of Attitudes toward Suffering

In some cases, caregivers may deny patients' suffering because increasing numbers of people are defining themselves as victims and as sufferers (Amato, 1990). They call for attention, resources, and compassion for conditions that were once regarded as the vicissitudes of life or a consequence of one's own behavior. Alcoholism, for instance, is a condition that was once considered to be the result of willful misconduct. In the United States, it is now usually regarded as a disease whose victims, now viewed as patients, require therapy and compassion. Today's inclusive definitions of suffering may be overwhelming to clinicians with limited access to resources, who then respond by "turning off" all patients' suffering.

Inattention to suffering is also related to the perspective that many present-day health-care professionals have of their mission—to cure patients with the application of scientific knowledge and techniques. The underlying perspective that disease has natural causes differed from earlier viewpoints that disease has supernatural sources (Lindberg, 1992). For example, the traditional Christian outlook, discussed in Chapter 4, was attentive to the diseases of the body and equally concerned with the accompanying anguish of the spirit. This view of the treatment of pathology recognized that physical disease was enmeshed in distinctly human qualities, such as the ability to grow spiritually through the experience of illness. Both patients and their caregivers regarded suffering either as the just consequence of one's own acts, and therefore to be endured, or as part of God's plan to be accepted with the promise of a better existence in eternity. In either case, suffering had a religious and culturally defined interpretation.

Supernatural perspectives prior to the development of science-based medicine are found also in some of the myths of classical civilizations, which depicted the sufferings of wounded heroes. These myths were replaced in the European theocratic society of the Middle Ages (5th to 15th centuries). In this age characterized by faith, the most persistent and influential institution was the Christian church, which taught how people should live. God was accepted as the final authority, and all life, including illness and suffering, were viewed as His realm (Tarnas, 1991); therefore, disease of the body and anguish of the soul were within God's domain and that of His healers.

SECULAR EXPLANATIONS FOR DISEASE

People began to challenge the unity of the body and spirit, however, when Arabic translations of ancient Greek physicians' writings became available in the 11th and 12th centuries (Lindberg, 1992). As medicine moved into the medieval university and came into contact with academic disciplines, explanations of diseases became more natural and theoretical. Secular explanations of phenomena gradually replaced those of God's revelations (Gordon, 1959). Those espousing secular interpretations were called humanists because they focused their interest on humans and their capacity to reason, and they began to question God as the single ultimate authority (Perry et al., 1985). Consequently, religious explanations of disease and suffering began to recede.

The beginnings of scientific inquiry and achievement evolved during the following years (Tarnas, 1991). Gradually, the human body was perceived as a part of matter, which could be studied by means of valued scientific methods. The idea developed that the body could be repaired much like a machine through the application of reason and growing scientific knowledge. Suffering was associated with the mind, which was not matter (Lindeboom, 1978); thus, suffering was excluded from the domain of science and became the responsibility of religion and philosophy. Because modern health care grew out of the scientific tradition, not religion and philosophy, attention to the machine-like body became the paramount concern in patient care. Separation of the body from the mind and spirit, where suffering is thought to exist, is the dominant perspective in much of health care today. Many clinicians, whose primary education is in the sciences, and health-care systems, which are intent on furnishing reimbursable services and eliciting demonstrable outcomes of health care, do not pay attention to suffering.

The suffering of patients is denied, not only because of caregiver fatigue and the sense that health care's mission does not properly include attention to suffering, but also because of clinicians' frustration when they *do* attempt to understand the phenomenon of suffering and to find guidelines for relieving it or helping patients bear it. The lack of scholarship about suffering in patient care is reflected in the fact that major health-care texts and bibliographic data bases, such as *Medline,* contain few citations for suffering. Those that do exist tend to equate suffering with physiological pain or to treat it as an indicator of disease or a secondary focus or illness. In view of the stated historical perspective, this finding is not surprising.

Accountability for Care of Sufferers

Suffering has not been abolished. It needs to be studied, understood, prevented, and alleviated, just as in past centuries communicable diseases needed to be investigated, prevented, and treated. The care of ill persons who suffer begins with recapturing interest in suffering and incorporating knowledge and understanding about it into today's biological model of health-care practice. Alleviating suffering demands that health-care professionals be *accountable* for its identification, prevention, understanding, and relief or management. Addressing patients' suffering is not a nicety; it is a critical standard of care for all settings in which patient services are furnished. Arguably, relief of suffering is the *sine qua non* of excellent total health care.

THREE KEY QUESTIONS

To care for those who suffer, health-care professionals need to consider three key questions:

1. *What is suffering?*
   Although frequently described and depicted, suffering in illness has rarely been subjected to analysis. Characteristically, consideration of suffering is found in social and religious tenets and in the history of ideas that constitute a context for understanding its nature. For the individual, suffering is typified by common convictions, such as the belief that he or she is in imminent danger. Identifying these beliefs and associated feelings and their sources helps health-care professionals determine how individuals experience suffering and directs these clinicians' initial actions toward its prevention or alleviation.

2. *What is the impact of clinicians on suffering?*
   The evidence indicates that the health-care system and its personnel are capable of both causing unnecessary suffering and modifying or alleviating suffering.

3. *How can suffering be endured or relieved?*
   Certain personal attributes of the clinician are essential to the relief of suffering, and selected approaches are commonly successful. General characteristics and patterns of suffering are

cognitively discernible, both to the clinician and to the sufferer; yet, in each instance, suffering is always a unique personal experience perceived through an individual's own prism of cherished values and life history. In the next chapters, a definition of suffering and a depiction of its general nature will be developed.

SUMMARY

Although many physical disorders and accompanying distress can be relieved by science-based knowledge and competence, the human experience of illness is largely beyond the realm of science. Suffering may be encountered in disease, pain, and dying, and clinicians must seek to heal the person who suffers as well as to treat the pathology. Yet, health-care professionals may be inattentive to suffering because of identifiable perceptions or circumstances. Neglect may be related also to a lack of understanding concerning the nature of suffering, the manner in which patients experience it, or the means by which clinicians can either relieve it or help patients to better tolerate it.

PRECEPT FOR PRACTICE

Providing quality care for the ill mandates a familiarity with the nature and expression of suffering.

REFERENCES

Amato, J. (1990). *Victims and values: A history and theory of suffering.* New York: Greenwood Press.

Auden, W.H. (1945). *The collected poetry of W. H. Auden.* New York: Random House.

Baring-Gould, S. (1878). *The mystery of suffering.* London: Skeffington and Son.

Gordon, B. (1959). *Medieval and renaissance medicine.* New York: Philosophical Library.

Hamilton, E. (1942). *Mythology.* Boston: Little, Brown and Company.

Lindberg, D. (1992). *The beginnings of western science: The European scientific tradition in philosophical, religious and institutional context, 600 B.C. to A.D. 1450.* Chicago: University of Chicago Press.

Lindeboom, G.A. (1978). *Des Cartes and medicine.* Amsterdam: Radopi.

Perry, M., et al. (1985). *Western civilization: Ideas, politics and society.* Boston: Houghton-Mifflin.

Tarnas, R. (1991). *The passion of the western mind: Understanding ideas that have shaped our world view.* New York: Ballantine Books.

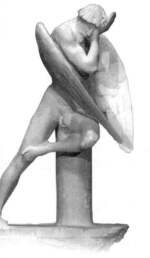

Chapter 2

What Is the Nature of Suffering?

To talk of suffering is not to talk of an academic problem but of the sheer bloody agonies of existence, of which all men are aware and most have some direct experience.

JOHN BOWKER (1975, P. 2)

There have been numerous efforts to define suffering that, while often thoughtful, give it limited substance. The following quote is an example:

> [Suffering is] that state of mind in which we wish violently or obsessively that our situation were otherwise. Such a state of mind involves memory and anticipation, the capacity to imagine alternatives, and (in man) a moral conscience (Hick 1966, p. 354).

The purpose of this chapter is to first establish a definition and description of the nature of suffering that is specific enough to be useful clinically and then to discuss sacred and secular views that shape the interpretation of suffering. Because no theory of suffering nor agreed on premises were discovered through a literature review, suffering's definition could not be established deductively; that is, from a common theory to the specifics. Rather, the explanation and distinctions of the general nature of suffering that are set forth were developed from the particulars. These specifics included findings from health-care and related literature and insights from literary depictions of suffering described throughout this work. The identified commonalities and patterns produced the definition and model that are presented later in this chapter. These abstractions are a product of inductive logical thought. The proposed structure of the phenomenon of suffering will require verification and modification through future study of human responses to illness; even so, suffering will likely remain more mysterious than logic alone can reveal.

Matrix of Suffering*

It first appears that suffering is formless, but on closer examination, health-care professionals as well as family members and friends are often able to determine what a patient most dreads and can thereby determine when suffering escalates in intensity. Such distinctions suggest that the elements that give suffering structure can be identified. Examination of available evidence suggests that suffering may be regarded as a matrix. It includes commonly manifest feelings that may be regarded as symptoms of suffering. Behind these feelings are threatened values and beliefs that give substance or essence to the symptoms.

Although most human beings have experienced suffering personally or vicariously, the term is vague and difficult to define; still it seems to be the best word to describe the state in which patients experience something that they would not choose ordinarily to endure. Other terms seem less adequate. *Pain* refers to a neurological sensation, although some authors use pain as a synonym for suffering. *Sorrow* and *grief* are associated typically with bereavement, one type of suffering. *Dolour* is primarily a literary term for suffering and is used uncommonly in health care. Etymologically, *passion* is a synonym that is related closely to suffering. It is derived from *pati*, which, as noted in the Preface, is also the Latin root for the word *patient*, one who suffers (Simpson & Werner, 1989). However, for Christians, *passion* has for centuries referred specifically to the suffering of Christ. Because it has taken on that singular meaning and is used principally in Christian theology, the term is not a usual part of health-care language. Because suffering appears to resist a narrow definition, a connotative definition may offer a more fruitful approach since features essential to the meaning can be included.

Suffering is characterized by its symptoms and underlying substance. **This work defines suffering as a syndrome of some duration, unique to the individual, involving a perceived relentless**

---

*Word etymology, definition, and analysis in this work are based on the following resources: Barnhart, R. (1995). *The Barnhart concise dictionary of etymology*; Glare, P.G.W. (Ed.) (1982). *Oxford Latin dictionary*; Gove, PG. (1993). *Webster's third new international dictionary of the English language*; Simpson, J.R. and Werner, E.S.C. (1989). *The Oxford English dictionary* and *Webster's dictionary of English usage*.

threat to one or more essential human values creating certain initially ominous beliefs and a range of related feelings. Suffering is the matrix in which fears, altered beliefs, and related emotions develop and in which they are embedded. Often the feelings that patients present, either verbally or nonverbally, first signal health professionals that suffering is present. The patient may appear upset, withdrawn, or overwhelmed. Gaining more patient information through collection of relevant data and verbal engagement can target the health-care professional's response and, at the same time, make the care more satisfying to patients because it is in accord with their particular emotional state and concerns about what the suffering signifies. It is both efficient and effective for subsequent care to attend to the patient's story by identifying the symptoms of the suffering, the substance of the patient's narrative, and the most pressing concerns expressed.

Intensity of Suffering

Clinicians are often unwilling or unable to evaluate the severity of the suffering expressed by patients. Perhaps this reluctance is related to the view that each person owns his or her suffering and that it cannot be compared to the suffering of others. In some cases, clinicians may simply be hesitant because they are unable to formulate a supportive response, or they may choose to be unresponsive to protect themselves from the personal pain that often follows engagement with a sufferer. However, the realities of clinical practice dictate that some differentiation can and should be made—if for no other reason than to allocate limited resources, one of which is professional time and attention.

Although a precise classification of the extent of suffering appears to exceed current knowledge, some further differentiation as to the degree of suffering seems possible. By analyzing, naming, and grouping the qualities that characterize the symptoms of suffering, four general categories of intensity emerge: distress, misery, anguish, and agony. The first category, distress, derives from the Latin *distringere,* which means to hinder or molest. For the patients who feel distress, conditions exist that produce strain and impede their normal life situations. These patients are troubled, disturbed, agitated, or worried. In earlier times, patients would have been said to be experiencing tribulation. Those who are distressed typically are able to hope that a more desirable state will be restored, and thus they are able at times to turn their attention to normal activities of living.

A second type of suffering, misery, is derived from the Latin word *miseria,* which means unhappiness or wretchedness. These persons are more deeply afflicted than those who are distressed. They are despondent and extremely unhappy. Their suffering occupies increased amounts of their attention, and they sense that returning to a more normal state will be difficult.

Some suffering is still more intense. The Latin word *angustia,* meaning difficulty or narrowness, is the source of the English word *anguish,* the third kind of suffering. Anguish is characterized by great suffering of the body or mind or both. In this state, patients fear that they will be unable to regain a normal life. They may have only brief respites from thinking about their suffering. In their anguish, as the word's derivation suggests, their existence narrows, and their focus is primarily on their suffering.

The most debilitating form of suffering is agony, from the Latin word *agonia,* which means a struggle. The struggle to survive suffering and its related conditions is excruciating to those who agonize, and the contest may be between life and death. It appears that extreme suffering or agony exists when patients' sustaining values are most challenged or even destroyed. The destruction of patients' life-organizing and guiding principles, moreover, seems to ruin patients' wholeness, damage their sense of connection with others, and rob them of meaning that nourishes life's quality. Suffering may be so extreme that it is expressed wordlessly as patients writhe and twist in their beds or become immobile. These patients may also feel *tormented,* a word etymologically associated with an instrument of torture, and they may wish for death. Nothing else exists for them but the unbearable suffering; it occupies their entire beings.

An expeditious general guide to evaluating the degree of suffering present was published by Barrell & Neimeyer (1975). The authors wrote that the magnitude of patients' feelings can be estimated by focusing on two questions. First, how much or how frequently do the patients think about their situations? If they think about them constantly, it is likely that intense suffering is present. Second, how significantly different is the current state of the patients from what they expected it to be? If the present situation is substantially different from a more positive expected state, the patient's level of suffering is likely to be severe. Patients' perceptions that the unfavorable situation cannot be altered further intensify the suffering; subsequently the patient often feels powerless to change its relentlessness.

Themes of Suffering

As the health care professional seeks to understand patients' suffering more fully and to address their needs more specifically, the knowledge of common themes and feelings associated with suffering and an understanding of threatened values related to the substance of suffering should assist the clinician to frame appropriate and sustaining responses. When patients' feelings are expressed, new underlying convictions emerge commonly and become truth for the patients. These themes or "new truths" evolve from the suffering and are associated with threats to sustaining values. Determining the nature of patients' beliefs before an illness enables clinicians to assist patients in their suffering and to project and interpret their behavior.

ISOLATION

One common theme in suffering is isolation. For example, those whose needs require nursing home care may be removed from their familiar communities and cherished friends to receive care and thus may feel banished. In one way or another, such patients express the belief, "I am alone." In their predicament, these sufferers feel set apart at a time when they most need to be in contact with others. They perceive themselves to be disconnected both from those who are not suffering and from their normal world. They may feel a little solitary (distress) or even abandoned (agony). The sustaining values that may be threatened are: (1) Being cared about for one's own sake is good, and (2) The ability to care for and about others is good (Van Wyk, 1990).

HOPELESSNESS

The second theme in suffering is hopelessness. The belief that "I am without hope" is embraced by the sufferer as true. Patients may feel that their problems bear down on them without solution. They may appear ineffective, confused, or despairing. These feelings may relate to the patient's inability to determine other ways of thinking about their situation or to choose other courses of action. For instance, those who lack financial resources may view obtaining needed care as impossible. The value that is threatened appears to be: Having alternative courses of action is good (Van Wyck, 1990).

VULNERABILITY

Suffering has other signatures. A third theme is that of vulnerability. The conviction of the sufferer is, "I am vulnerable to hurt." For example, patients may feel uneasy (distress) or dread (agony) that they will be harmed physically or emotionally while tolerating the side effects of aggressive chemotherapy. Patients may not only believe that they are susceptible to harm but also feel that other persons (sometimes caregivers) have the power to harm them. Consequently, they feel helpless and see the future as menacing. At its core, vulnerability threatens the value: It is good to exist and make full use of one's abilities (Van Wyck, 1990).

LOSS

A fourth theme of suffering is loss. While vulnerability involves concerns about future deprivation, loss more commonly entails something that has already been damaged. Patients believe, "I have experienced a great loss." The perceived sense of loss may result in temporary disadvantage (distress), or it may be related to decreased autonomy, bodily change, deprivation of good health, or loss of the former self such as may be experienced with quadriplegia. Losses that are interpreted by patients as significant may cause them to question what is sustaining in their lives, and loss of meaning can be agonizing. Loss challenges the value that: Having satisfying beliefs about one's place in the universe is good (Van Wyck, 1990). In some cases, feelings of vulnerability, loss, and meaninglessness are comingled.

The sense of loss takes myriad forms, some obvious and others less so. What the patient has been deprived of may be apparent from a situation like paralysis; however, the loss may also be symbolic. When a patient experiences a disability or impairment, the patient's suffering may be related not only to physical changes, but also to altered roles in the family or in the workplace or to other reasons. Soon after a loss, clinicians may relieve suffering by simply hearing the patient's lament, "I will never walk normally again." It is important to listen and understand that the patient ordinarily must encounter the suffering to begin healing. By acknowledging the loss verbally, the patient begins to accept its reality and opens the possibility of being comforted. Later work may involve exploring issues of meaning so that the patient is able to make sense of the loss and perhaps transcend it.

It is the duty of health-care professionals to attempt to recognize and address patients' feelings and the beliefs and values that underlie their suffering. Simply saying, "I know this is difficult for you" or "I can see that you are having a bad day" acknowledges the existence of suffering and penetrates the patient's solitary world, offering the presence of a compassionate companion in the suffering. Even in cases where no cure is possible, the patient can always be offered the fidelity of health-care professionals and the expectation that symptoms will be well managed.

The Quest for a Common Etiology

Because analysis suggests that some consistent themes are present in the manner in which suffering evolves and is presented, a common etiology may emerge. Studying suffering from various disciplinary perspectives, especially reviewing literary narratives of suffering, reiterates an essence captured in the German word *angst* because it encompasses in its meaning, dread, anxiety, and fear of the future. An ancient psalmist illustrates:

> I am terrified,
> and the terrors of death crush me.
> I am gripped by fear and trembling;
> I am overcome with horror.
> (PSALM 55, 4–5)

Concomitant with all suffering is some element of fear. Etymologically, the word *fear* is derived from the Old English *far* or *fare,* which means danger or disaster. Initiated by a sense of imminent danger from powers beyond one's control, fear often launches the process of suffering seen by clinicians, because the patient's world view and sometimes his or her very existence are threatened by the disease or the circumstances.

CHARACTERISTICS OF FEAR

It is unknown whether a perceived danger causes all suffering; however, it seems that when a patient senses a real or symbolic danger, fear follows, and suffering is likely to occur. The impending peril may be generic, precise, or vague. Taylor's research (1993) suggests that certain generic fears are very basic to the human condition and, if not universal, are widely held. He has defined these elemental fears as fear of mental incapacitation, death, and/or suffering. In illness, then, suffering could result from fear of suffering itself or of mental incapacity or of death as well as from causes unique to the individual. Although certain approaches to care described herein and elsewhere may prove helpful, it may be that suffering is so integral to humanness as to make removal of fears associated with patients' very being problematic.

Either precise or vague fears, in contrast to elemental generic fears, may be more amenable to definition and treatment. Specific fears may be protective when a real or perceived imminent danger can be avoided or, in some cases, alleviated. For example, a preoperative patient may be able to identify a fear of general anesthesia explicitly. If the fear is related to misconceptions, information may ameliorate the fear. In other cases, regional anesthesia may be an appropriate option, thus removing the cause of the specific fear.

A sense of general endangerment, however, results in a vague fear when a danger associated with his illness cannot be described with certainty, as when the patient feels that treatment options are equally unsatisfactory. Changes in thinking, behavior, and even physiology may be related to a perceived or generalized evil that menaces the patient (Hodiamont, 1991). Reactions are most foreboding when one or more of patients' basic personal values that are central to their sense of coherence are threatened. When endangered, the familiar self may be damaged when illness and the associated distress prevent patients from living and acting in accord with their life values. Highly independent and self-sufficient patients, for example, frequently have difficulty accepting needed care.

Fear, accompanied by powerlessness and uncertainty, has been portrayed as suffering. Tuan (1979) noted that a person who experiences threats has two sensations: "One is the fear of the imminent collapse of his world and the approach of death . . .. The other is a sense of personalized evil, the feeling that the hostile force, whatever its specific manifestation, possesses evil as suffering" (p. 7). According to the author, a fearsome event initiates an alarm followed by a sense of dread about the future, especially when the menace is so vague that it prevents action.

IDENTIFYING FEAR

While it is not known whether a common etiology for all suffering exists, the foregoing postulates that a perceived fearful danger is the agent that potentially initiates suffering. Fear threatens a patient's important, sustaining values, resulting in feelings that can be detected by astute clinicians. If the patient's values are enduring and overcome the threat, suffering may be prevented, modified, or better tolerated.

However, if the values are overwhelmed and the patient anticipates an uncontrollable negative outcome, then dread ensues and suffering escalates. Such patients suffer because their situations seem to be or are out of their control, and appropriate action, therefore, cannot be identified. Health-care professionals need to listen attentively to patients' descriptions of suffering to identify their fears and their sustaining values as well as their feelings. For example, patients who fear an uncertain future may be rendered powerless by paternalistic health-care professionals who have not identified or communicated care alternatives.

Because fear is often suppressed or disguised, the most significant question to ask of the sufferer may be, **"What is most frightening (or of greatest concern) to you about this situation?"** Many patients will answer this question very specifically and feel relieved to have been asked. Given the opportunity to express feelings aloud, patients will often find answers within themselves. Answers arrived at in this way are likely to be more satisfying than those suggested by others.

The answer to the foregoing question often reveals the major source of difficulty for a particular patient. For example, a patient who has developed hemiplegia may reply, "I am of no use." What is threatened by his disease is his choice of determining how he will function and control his mode of being. Consequently, he feels hopeless, which may be reflected in feelings that range from discouragement (distress) to total despair (agony). In some cases, it is necessary to help the patient identify the value that is at risk. Because greater fear and powerlessness may be evident when patients are unable to identify the value that is in jeopardy, helping patients to articulate what is important to them or at least name their terrors may identify their threatened values and may prove helpful. Struggling to understand what patients think suffering is and discovering how suffering has placed something of value at risk for the patient enables health-care professionals to respond to the needs of the sufferer. As David Morris (1996) summarized, "The need to hear a voice is rarely stronger than when a patient endures suffering" (p. 32).

A Model of Suffering

The foregoing analysis is intended to sensitize the health-care professional's ability to discover and begin to comprehend the sufferer's experience. These concepts will be developed more fully in the following chapters. Identifying the elements can expand the number and the quality of the clinician's response repertoire. The model that follows visually represents the foregoing discussion about the substance, beliefs, and feelings that unfold in the matrix of suffering. The model proposes a pattern to enhance understanding and to guide health-care professionals in patient care to:

1. Relate patients' feelings to the more complex phenomenon of suffering
2. Recognize some beliefs that may underlie emotions
3. Identify the threatened values that support the beliefs
4. Estimate the intensity of the suffering
5. Establish priorities for intervention and care among a group of patients
6. Respond in accord with the patient's perceived state

The model is offered with the caution that an analysis and depiction of suffering may not represent a particular individual's experience of suffering because such a model is inherently reductionist; that is, it simplifies the complex. The sufferer's life experience and understanding of his situation is ultimately the best guide. An analysis suggests, but does not decree, what suffering is for a unique human being; however, once the common symptoms of suffering and the threatened values are identified, many clinicians are then able to empathize, communicate, and apply therapeutic modalities to relieve suffering or to sustain patients in it (see Fig. 2–1).

Perspectives on Suffering

Developing answers to the question, "What is suffering?" is germane to the goal of relieving suffering or at least helping patients to better bear it. Understanding suffering requires the health professional to be cognizant of both current and historical beliefs about suffering along with important background factors such as culture and demographic characteristics that are beyond the scope of this work. While common characteristics of suffering can be identified, suffering, as indicated previously, is ultimately configured uniquely by the patient.

The beliefs that constitute suffering are often the most significant contextual issue. Patients' perspectives may or may not be shared by other sufferers or by their families or caregivers. When the patient's sense about what suffering is, why it exists, what its personal significance may be, and how it should be borne are not shared by the clinician, it is incumbent on the health-care professional to elicit the meaning of suffering for the patient and honor the patient's convictions. Uncommonly the patient invites exploration of those

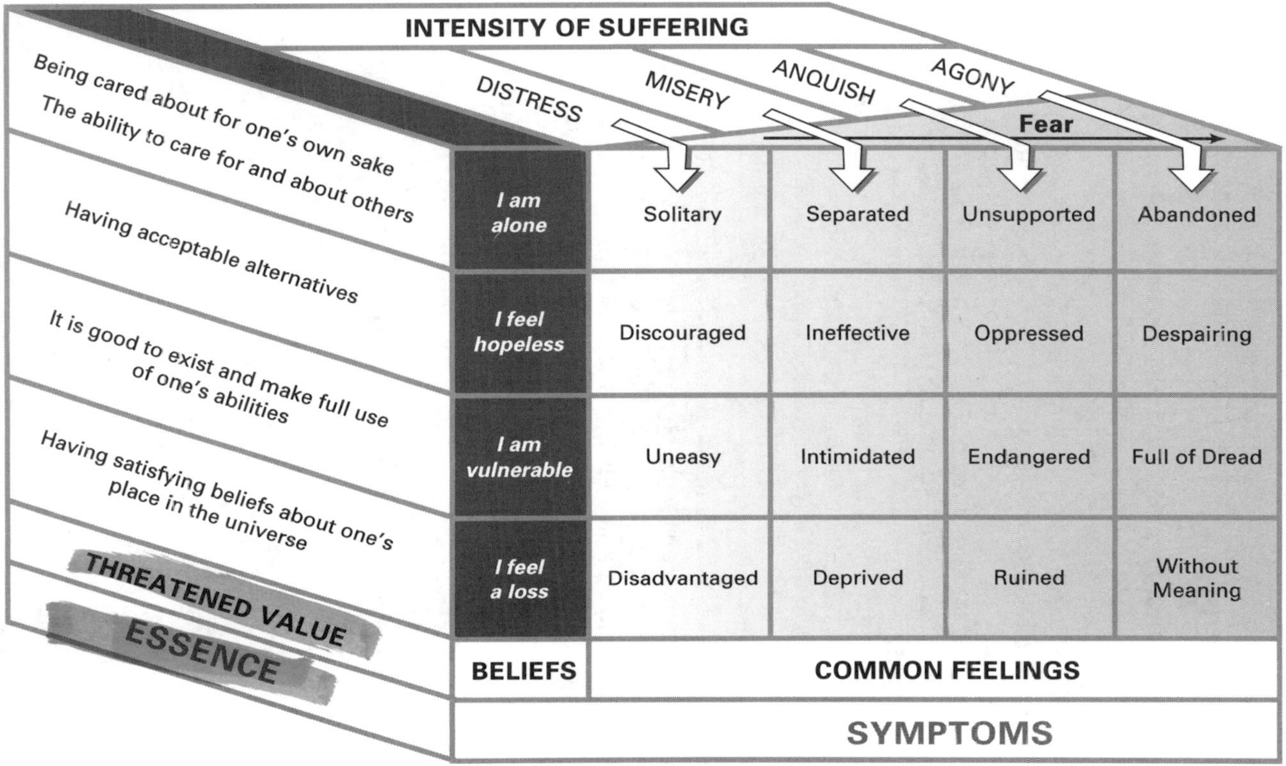

FIGURE 2–1. Proposed Model of Suffering.

differences, but if asked, the clinician may offer his or her honest perceptions, without implying judgment.

SUPERNATURAL BELIEFS

Basically two general perspectives on the nature of suffering exist. One view may be defined as supernatural, religious, or theistic, while the other may be described as natural, secular, or nontheistic. A contemporary example of how supernatural beliefs impact suffering is the commonly held, often-stated view of the AIDS epidemic. The emergence of AIDS in the homosexual community was sometimes proclaimed as a rightful scourge of God on sinners. This conviction explains, in part, why efforts to obtain resources for AIDS patients when the disease was first identified met with limited success. The underlying belief that these patients should rightfully endure their suffering as a just retribution for their sins made securing even meager resources difficult in the early years of the epidemic.

Punishment

Viewing suffering as a punishment is hardly a new idea. Religion provided early civilizations with interpretations of good and of evil that included suffering (Perry, et al., 1985). For the most part, suffering was regarded as largely inevitable, but, in some cases, it could be avoided by appeasing the gods (Amato, 1990). Even before writing was established, some of the myths of classical civilizations set forth the idea that transgression of the will of the gods resulted in punishment and suffering.

One of the Greek myths that has survived is that of the Titan Prometheus, a primeval deity (Guerber, 1943). It was Prometheus who, against the edict of Zeus, gave humans the gift of fire, which represented art, commerce, and civilization, thus making humans different from other creatures and elevating their status. When mortals then began to neglect the gods, Zeus penalized them by depriving them of this gift. Prometheus, however, was compassionate and restored the fire. Consequently, Zeus punished Prometheus by chaining him to the peak of Mount Caucasus where a huge eagle gnawed at his liver every day inflicting horrible pain. According to the legend, the liver grew back each night so that Prometheus's torture persisted for centuries until Hercules killed the eagle and finally freed the suffering Prometheus (Hamilton, 1942).

In *Prometheus Bound,* the dramatist Aeschylus (525/524 to 456/455 BCE [before the common era]) had Prometheus declare his suffering to be a punishment for his crime, however undeserved.

I dared do it, I delivered man
From death and steep destruction. Such the crime
For which I pay with these fell agonies,
Painful to suffer, pitiful to see.
For pitying man in preference to myself
I am debarred from pity; and thus I stand
Tortured, to Zeus a spectacle of shame
(THOMPSON, TRANS. 1979, P. 67).

Clinicians will observe in this excerpt that some of their patients share certain beliefs of this ancient myth, namely: (1) suffering is a form of punishment for a transgression, (2) suffering must be endured stoically, (3) suffering is associated with pain, and (4) suffering may serve a higher purpose. The myth, moreover, makes clear to health-care professionals that suffering may have more than one etiology, although only one cause may be readily apparent. Prometheus suffered from unrelieved physical pain, but he also suffered from the injustice of a punishment inflicted because he had treated humans with compassion. From Prometheus, to the self-punishing Flagellants of the Middle Ages (Reisman, 1936), to modern AIDS patients, suffering continues to be linked to punishment.

Incomprehensible

Although some patients believe that their suffering is a form of punishment and may accept it as the will of God, others regard their suffering as incomprehensible. Health-care professionals, too, wrestle with the question of why the innocent suffer. Caring for a young person dying of cancer or trying to comfort a family after a fatal automobile accident challenges some deeply held religious beliefs and understandings of justice.

The age-old perception that suffering is an impenetrable mystery persists today. Some early Jewish writers sustained the view that suffering is the consequence of sin while at the same time they challenged that perspective, as found in the story of Job in the Hebrew *Bible (Old Testament.)* Job was clearly a righteous man; still, he suffered as the result of a skin disease, the loss of his wealth, and the death of his children. Throughout his ordeal, however, Job sustained his faith in God (YHWH)[†] and was, in the end, blessed. Religious scholars have long studied and commented on the story of Job. Often the narrative is interpreted to mean that although suffering may not be

---

[†]In Judaism, the names of God may be proper names or represent the nature of God. The most frequently used name of God in the Old Testament is YHWH, which is pronounced Yahweh or Yahaweh (Singer, 1905).

comprehended in the present, it will be understood in time. For some patients, suffering is seen as a test of faith as it was for Job.

It is not difficult to recognize the view in present patient-care situations that suffering is difficult to grasp with the rational mind. For instance, survivors often ask, "Why did he die so young? There was so much more good for him to do." Those who seek to comfort may respond, "We cannot always understand God's plan." The popularity of the book *When Bad Things Happen to Good People,* written by Rabbi Harold Kushner in 1981, confirmed with its popularity the struggle of many persons with suffering's incomprehensibility. Publication of this book, in fact, was the outcome of Rabbi Kushner's own efforts to make sense of the suffering and death of his young son.

Meaningful

While some patients view suffering as punishment and others regard it as a test of faith or as unfathomable, still others find greater significance beyond the experience of suffering. The quest is summarized often in the question, "Why?" which may be accompanied by feelings of despair, hopelessness, frustration, or anger. In the process, beliefs may be discarded, modified, or affirmed, and the suffering may be relieved, better endured, or transcended. Transcending suffering—that is, placing it in a larger context—is somewhat analogous to focusing on the joy of the child-to-be during the pain of labor. For many people, transcendence involves religious beliefs that link them to the security of that which is everlasting and beyond their current travails.

It is in the very character of religion to attend to universals and to ascribe significance to experience. The nature of suffering and how it should be borne may be culturally determined and is addressed by religions frequently; it is central in Buddhism and Christianity. For the Buddhist, awareness of suffering is a stimulus to learning and spiritual development. Suffering is regarded as an illusion that can be surmounted through detachment and discipline. In Christianity, suffering is associated with the sacrifice of Christ that is believed to lead to the redemption of sinners (Heitman, 1992) and to restoring the sinner's relationship with God (Amato, 1990). The relationship of specific beliefs to suffering is explored more fully in a later chapter.

Health-care professionals often encounter patients who are struggling to go beyond their suffering or who have already transcended it, although that particular term is heard infrequently. After trauma or a significant illness, patients may report that they became more understanding of, sensitive to, and caring about the misfortune of others through their own anguish. Former patients sometimes become active in philanthropic work or in support groups that assist persons in unfortunate circumstances. Health-care professionals themselves often have been motivated to become providers of care through an experience with illness and suffering—their own or that of others. The desire to help others frequently has its genesis in personal or vicarious suffering. The adolescent with leukemia who elects a health-related career or the cancer support groups that ably and compassionately serve others who are afflicted are examples of this phenomenon. Thus suffering sometimes can be transcended and become a means for growth wherein humans discover a greater or universal meaning or purpose, even though the suffering may persist.

Secular Beliefs

NATURAL PHENOMENA

Supernatural perspectives on suffering are not embraced by all persons. For some patients, secular views can also explain, help them endure, or give significance to their suffering. One secular perspective on suffering developed in the West when the theistic Christian explanation of the Middle Ages shifted to a profound faith in human reason, and science was crystallized by Newtonian physics in the 17th century (Tarnas, 1991). Reliance on logic and science began with Renee Decartes (1596–1650 CE [common era]) who asserted that "truth" could be discovered by the application of reason rather than by God's revelation of truth alone (Burns et al., 1984). This view ushered in the cosmology of the 16th and 17th centuries and was affirmed by the publication of *Mathematical Principals* (*Philosophae Naturalis Principa Mathematica*) by Sir Isaac Newton (Newton, 1686). *Principa* described the laws of motion and is considered by some scholars to be the greatest scientific achievement ever (Burns, 1984). It profoundly changed ways of thinking thereafter.

More than 2 centuries later, clinicians observe that many of their patients accept illness as due to natural causes or express an overwhelming belief that science will have the answers to their impaired health and, by extension, will alleviate their suffering. The methods of science have relieved or prevented much suffering by conquering disease and furnishing methods for cures or effective management of symptoms. Science and its methods that seek to achieve objective certainty, however, often disappoint patients and clinicians alike when the goal is to relieve suffering itself. Technology can even distance the health-care professional from the patient when data become more important than the patient's experience (Reiser, 1992).

SOCIAL PHENOMENA

Another secular view, sometimes shared by religious persons, attributes suffering largely to family or community causes. Sufferers often regard themselves as victims of the state or of society. This view can be identified in many cases among persons who seek treatment for substance abuse. As they relate their illness histories to health-care professionals, some persons link their afflictions largely to dysfunctional families, spousal abuse, poverty, or other social problems. The belief that suffering can be addressed through political or social reform can be traced to Jeremy Bentham (1748–1832) (Amato, 1990). Continuing the thinking of The Age of Reason, Bentham was optimistic that the state could solve human problems, including suffering of various types. For example, social reform measures implemented in London in the 1840s and 1850s, when deplorable living conditions of the poor were discovered, exemplified this optimistic view (Metz, 1991). While we may assume that these measures were initiated by compassion, as a practical matter, members of the middle and upper classes acted expeditiously because they also feared infection with communicable diseases associated with the unhygienic living conditions of the poor.

The optimism of the 18th-century Enlightenment view that humans and social systems could be perfected remained influential and was evident during the mid-20th century in the goals of The Great Society. Established under President Lyndon Johnson, numerous programs were initiated based on the assumption that life's difficulties could be eliminated or at least improved through funding social initiatives. Some of these programs, such as Medicare, were designed to furnish illness care for elderly adults and were even perceived to relieve its companion, suffering. In Amato's (1990) view, however, the unbridled optimism of The Great Society, which equated unhappiness with suffering, resulted in unrealistic expectations of social programs to relieve suffering so defined.

Existential Views

There is an additional view of suffering that is usually secular but may not be wholly so. It is associated with those persons who assert that suffering, and indeed any human condition, can be defined neither by science nor religion nor society. Those who hold this view assert that the reasons for suffering are unknown. For them, the world is an uncertain place; therefore, they rely on the analysis of their own existential experience for guidance, particularly in crisis situations. When health-care professionals interact with such persons, they may discover that some patients hold nihilistic views, rejecting or at least doubting established interpretations of suffering offered by religion or science or the culture, although they usually accept science-based care for physical disorders.

COUNSELING PERSPECTIVES

Patients who hold secular views of the nature of suffering offer particular challenges to clinicians. While interactions with persons who hold supernatural beliefs can draw on identifiable religious truths, caring for sufferers with secular perspectives has fewer touchstones; therefore, it is more difficult. In general, patients with a secular outlook place a greater value on self-determination and the opportunity to create their meaning in light of their own unique journeys through life. They share with religious patients the need to be listened to nonjudgmentally and empathically. Clinicians must attempt to assist all patients who are receptive to discover some significance in their distress that gives continued purpose to living beyond the circumstances of the suffering. The understandings of the nature of suffering are many and complex as are the efforts to comprehend them. But in undertaking this responsibility, health-care professionals may gain greater expertise and, even more important, the satisfaction of providing comfort to those who suffer.

SUMMARY _____

Health-care professionals must be accountable for preventing, detecting, relieving, and helping patients to endure their suffering. This responsibility may be inadequately fulfilled because the treatment of pathology alone often takes precedence over the patient's experience of illness. Clinical encounters with sufferers leave some health-care professionals uncertain about how to proceed. Knowing what patients believe about the nature of suffering and their experiences of it prepares health-care professionals to respond. Some understandings about suffering have religious foundations while others are based on secular or personal philosophies.

Suffering is unique to the individual, but analysis does suggest some common attributes. First, suffering appears to be initiated by a perceived danger that elicits fear. It is often characterized by beliefs related to a sense of isolation, hopelessness, vulnerability, and loss that the patient regards as real, perhaps not subject to change, although relief may be possible. The sufferer's beliefs are expressed in feelings of varying intensity that constitute the symptoms of suffering. Some threatened values are suggested but may vary among cultures, among individuals within a culture, among belief systems or philosophies, and according to individual life experiences. Sensitivity to the patterns and dynamics that signal the presence of suffering is essential to the work of the clinician, which begins with identifying a patient's convictions about suffering. Suffering will be further described in the next chapter from the point of view of the sufferer so that health-care professionals are positioned to see, hear, and relieve it.

PRECEPT FOR PRACTICE

Recognizable signs, patterns, and dynamics of suffering signal its existence and provide the foundation for initiating care.

REFERENCES

Amato, J. (1990). *Victims and values: A history and theory of suffering.* New York: Greenwood Press.

Barnhart, R. (Ed.). (1995). *The Barnhart concise dictionary of etymology.* New York: Harper-Collins.

Barrell, J., & Neimeyer, R. (1975). A mathematical formula for the psychological control of suffering. *Journal of Pastoral Counseling, 10,* 60–67.

Bowker, J. (1970). *Problems of suffering in religions of the world.* Cambridge: Cambridge University Press.

Burns, E.M., et al. (1984). *Western civilizations: Their history and their culture.* New York: W.W. Norton Company.

Glare, P.G.W. (Ed.). (1982). *Oxford Latin dictionary.* New York: Oxford University Press.

Good news Bible: Today's English version (1992). Nashville, Tenn.: Thomas Nelson Publishers.

Gove, P. (Ed.), and the Merriam Webster editorial staff (1993). *Webster's third new international dictionary of the English language, unabridged.* Springfield, Mass.: Merriam Webster.

Guerber, H.A. (1943). *The myths of Greece and Rome.* London: George Harrap and Company, Ltd.

Hamilton, E. (1942). *Mythology.* Boston: Little, Brown and Company.

Heitman, E. (1992). The influence of values and culture in response to suffering. In P.L. Stark & J.P. McGovern (Eds.), *The hidden dimension of illness: Human suffering* (pp. 81–105). New York: NLN Press.

Hick, J. (1966). *Evil and the God of love.* New York: Harper and Row.

Hodiamont, P. (1991). How normal are anxiety and fear? *International Journal of Social Psychiatry 37*, 43–50.

Kushner, H. (1981). *When bad things happen to good people.* New York: Schoken Books.

Metz, N. (1991). Discovering a world of suffering: Fiction and rhetoric of sanitary reform, 1840–1860. *Nineteenth Century Contexts, 15*(1), 65–79.

Morris, D. (1996). About suffering: Voice, genre and moral community. *Daedalus, 125*(1), 23–45.

Newton, I. (1686/1962). *Mathematical Principles* (A. Motte, trans., (1729); Revised, F. Cajori, 1940). New York: Greenwood Press.

Perry, M. (1985). *Western civilization: Ideas, politics and society.* Boston: Houghton-Mifflin.

Reiser, S. (1992). Technologic environments as causes of suffering: The ethical context. In P. Stark & J. McGovern (Eds.), *The hidden dimension of illness: Human suffering* (pp. 43–52). New York: NLN Press.

Reisman, D. (1936). *The story of medicine in the middle ages.* New York: Paul Hoeber, Inc.

Simpson, J.R., & Werner, E.S.C. (Eds.). (1989). *The Oxford English dictionary.* New York: Oxford University Press.

Singer, I. (Ed.). (1905). *Jewish encyclopedia.* Volume IX, Names of God. London: Funk and Wagnalls Company.

Tarnas, R. (1991). *The passion of the western mind.* New York: Ballantine Books.

Taylor, S. (1993). The structures of fundamental fears. *Journal of Behavior Therapy and Experimental Psychiatry 24*(4), 289–99.

Thompson, G. (Ed./Trans.). (1979). *Aeschylus: The Prometheus bound.* New York: Arnco Press.

Tuan, Y.F. (1979). *Landscape of fear.* New York: Pantheon Books.

Van Wyk, R. (1990). *Introduction to ethics.* New York: St. Martin's Press.

Webster's dictionary of English usage (1989). Springfield, Mass.: Merriam-Webster.

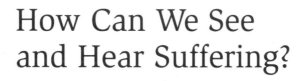

Chapter 3

How Can We See and Hear Suffering?

Perhaps we should seek forgiveness for the neglect we have demonstrated in the past and continue to demonstrate when we fail to support and feel for the suffering humanity that continues to cry out for our help.

LEONARD LIEGNER (1986–87, P. 93)

Although health-care professionals may treat pathology successfully, their patients' humanness may be injured by the suffering that accompanies their illness and sometimes by its treatment modalities. These wounds may be neither visible nor scientifically verifiable, but they exist and may heal slowly or not at all. The preceding chapters discussed the features that signal that suffering is present. Although it is important to identify these symptoms and characteristics, true understanding is more than cognitive. In this chapter, reasons for the denial of suffering are identified and suffering is examined through the perspective of several relevant disciplines.

Myths and Perceptions that Support the Denial of Suffering

Health-care professionals, either consciously or unconsciously, may choose to avoid and deny suffering. Even when circumstances permit involvement, some professionals may limit contact with sufferers as much as possible and enter the sickroom only to perform technical procedures. Others appear to be more available to the patient but insulate themselves with a professional demeanor that distances them from the suffering patient. Frequently both caregivers and patients share beliefs or myths that support denial, a condition that accompanies the avoidance of suffering.

MYTH NO. 1: GOOD HEALTH IS DURABLE

A myth, common among young persons, is that their robust health will be continuous. When patients become acutely ill or a condition cannot be improved by further treatment, the myth is shattered. Even when the physical condition can be well managed, patients may suffer from intrinsic concerns about the illness or from inexperience with adversity and lack of personal resources with which to cope with misfortune. Their situations are like that described by George Eliot (1859/1917) in *Adam Bede:*

> For there is no despair so absolute as that which comes with the first moments of our first great sorrow, when we have not yet known what it is to have suffered and healed, to have despaired and recovered hope (p. 322).

This observation may be applied not only to patients but also to health-care professionals who have not encountered suffering in their families or in their own lives or who have not met suffering with a patient or even experienced suffering vicariously through a liberal education. It explains why caring for a patient of the same age, sex, social group, educational level, or life circumstances is often very difficult for the clinician. Such inexperience with suffering may lead a clinician to adopt a style of practice that avoids dealing with patients' suffering.

MYTH NO. 2: SCIENCE ALWAYS RESTORES HEALTH

"Science will cure suffering" is the second myth that contributes to neglect or denial of suffering. Science cures some diseases, manages others, and also moderates the accompanying physical symptoms successfully. In some cases, the application of the techniques of medical science not only cures the disease but also relieves the suffering that originates in the physical disorder. In other situations, a deeper suffering remains in spite of the best science. In fact, relief of troublesome physical symptoms may afford patients the opportunity to contemplate their nonphysical suffering (Gregory, 1994).

Illness can alter a patient's world profoundly and engender suffering unrelated to the pathology. The disorder of the body may restrict or make impossible the patient's customary lifestyle. It may forever change long-established roles and relationships with family members and with the larger community. Illness may end work, productivity, and financial security and thereby cause suffering.

Perhaps more importantly, suffering may persist because it has damaged or destroyed the meanings that have structured a patient's life or made the old meanings inapplicable to a new situation. The sufferer may doubt or become alienated from those beliefs and values that shaped his goals and became his anchors before the illness. For some religious persons, for instance, suffering may transform an ever-present and loving creator to a distant and impersonal god who inflicts punishment unjustly.

For other patients, the belief in a rational world is no longer suited to the suffering associated with random and inexplicable tragedy. Undesired changes in that which is central to existence may make patients feel as if their lives have been shattered. A patient's suffering becomes so profound that there may be ". . . a rupture between his condition and the image of the whole by which he is bound to life and the world" (Rawlinson, 1986, p. 48). A positivist view of science is not helpful in such situations because it is inattentive to those human concerns that produce suffering; it does not encompass the total existential context of the pathology or the person who suffers.

The myth that science can relieve suffering unfailingly is sustained by three perceptions that health-care professionals and patients may share:

1. *Suffering may be understood and treated with the same type of clear protocols that are associated with the science-based treatment of disease.*
   Although this methodology proves effective for relieving disease-related problems, suffering is of a different order. Some health-care professionals are unprepared to employ alternative strategies or to persist when there are no immediate results and suffering continues.

2. *Suffering can be wholly relieved without investment of the self.*
   In some cases, to be sure, suffering related to pathology can be ameliorated by the knowledgeable, direct intervention of competent health-care professionals. More often, however, suffering is addressed through a human encounter that blurs the distinction between the person who is the health-care professional and the person who is the patient. This encounter may seem threatening to patients who are not introspective and to health-care professionals who have been educated to "be objective" in their patient-care activities. For both participants, the territory is uncharted. Accustomed to predicting recovery trajectories with critical paths and to relying on reasoned diagnoses and treatment protocols, health-care professionals feel vulnerable in the chaos of

suffering where few familiar landmarks exist and where they must share the suffering to some degree to address it.

3. *Finally, there is the perception and expectation—often unrealistic—that suffering can be fully eradicated.*
   Some suffering seems to be inevitable, and, in certain cases, the health-care professional can only hope to sustain patients and to support their efforts to transcend it. Other suffering may only be modified but not relieved in the time available. What is always unconscionable is that some patients suffer because health-care professionals fail to *prevent* suffering when they are in a position to do so. Health-care professionals must always remain committed to preventing and alleviating suffering and to providing palliative care when suffering cannot be relieved satisfactorily.

MYTH NO. 3: SUFFERING CAN BE CURED

Another myth that undermines attention to suffering is that it can be relieved quickly. Some harried health-care professionals become impatient when compassionate care of the sufferer reveals itself to require extended attention rather than an episodic intervention. At its core, caring for a sufferer is a courageous act that involves understanding what suffering is for a patient and applying knowledge and care guided by that understanding. Even when the clinician does not comprehend fully the nature of suffering for a particular patient, the struggle to understand it is likely to be perceived as caring by the patient (Sarason, 1985). Ultimately, it is the patient who determines the nature of the caring required; there are no standardized protocols. The model of suffering described earlier, however, may furnish guidance for the health-care professional to open communication and to initiate care.

MYTH NO. 4: EASING SUFFERING REQUIRES ACTION

The belief that a health-care professional must always "do something" to relieve suffering may interfere with its relief. On occasion, care of suffering may require "only" presence and attentive silence. Sometimes suffering renders a patient silent because it comes suddenly or is very intense. Patients may be so overwhelmed, fragile, or fearful that they are unable to articulate their suffering. In such situations, health-care professionals—particularly those who have not experienced suffering personally—may feel uncomfortable, and in their unease, chatter. Experienced clinicians know, however, that

attention and empathic listening offer relief without words—
acknowledging and validating the suffering. Further comfort may be
offered by appropriate touch, thereby making the patient feel less
isolated by reaching into his miserable world. Although caring may be
expressed silently, a mutuality can be created. As described by Griffith
(1970), the process is somewhat mystical. He writes:

> Experience with the mystery (of suffering) takes one beyond the
> realm of ideas and produces finally a kind of muteness or at least a
> reticence to express in words the solace that can only be expressed
> by an attitude of union with the sufferer (p. 26).

Disciplinary Perspectives That Illuminate Suffering

When health-care professionals become aware of suffering and choose
to be accountable for responding to suffering, perspectives and skills
from various disciplines can aid them. Some disciplines bring the
clinicians closer to the actual suffering of an individual than can be
furnished by a cognitive understanding of the configuration of
suffering described previously.

BEHAVIORAL AND SOCIAL SCIENCES

Behavioral science, for example, grapples with how patients cope
with suffering. Through various therapeutic approaches, psychology
attends to emotion, thought, and action. A behaviorist view, for
instance, emphasizes that patients examine their experiences,
expectations, and environments in relation to their suffering, and then
discover and incorporate new modes of action into more effective
behavior (Fordyce, 1988). When a patient learns more competent
interaction skills, for instance, suffering associated with loneliness in
chronic illness may be relieved, reducing the need for intervention or
support by professionals. Developmental approaches to psychology
attempt to understand how patients have established beliefs or ways
of coping with distress that influence a current situation. Behavioral
patterns, such as helplessness, that the clinician identifies may enable
patients to see their situations more clearly and thereby ease their
suffering.

The social sciences explore the impact of a social group or
environment, the way people define illness, the manner in which they
seek care, the norms that specify how suffering is expressed, and the

responses to illness that are appropriate. For example, persons who are stoic when they experience pain may receive little care or attention in a culture that responds to expressiveness.

The behavioral and social sciences furnish theories and methods to study specific problems and phenomena associated with suffering. They also include skills and generate instruments or strategies that are useful in defining or resolving identified problems. Scholars in these disciplines, however, have rarely studied suffering as an entity and tend to focus on important but more narrowly defined concerns such as coping or the sick role.

RELIGION AND PHILOSOPHY

In contrast, religious scholars and philosophers have directed their studies more broadly. Typically, they focus on the ultimate questions or realities of which suffering is a part. A central question is, "What is the significance of suffering?" Such questions may involve formulating an explanation for the existence of suffering, but often a specific justification cannot be determined for an individual case. Dependent on the particular philosophical or theological framework, comprehension of suffering may be related to understanding good and evil, or suffering may be attributed to a random happening. Suffering may also be regarded as sent by God as a test of strength or as simply incomprehensible. In individual cases, therefore, suffering may be a fact, problem, or stimulus for growth, or it may require resignation and acceptance.

Each discipline furnishes useful perspectives or tools; however, the clinician must remember that a discipline is an abstraction that represents a more complex human phenomenon. Patients who suffer do not fit into neat disciplinary boxes. Suffering is a human experience that may have physical, social, emotional, *and* spiritual aspects. Theory should inform and guide but not constrain clinicians. Bear theory humbly into the presence of a suffering human being.

Seeing Suffering through Literature

The study of literature, including religious literature, together with psychotherapy and art, provides even greater insight into individual suffering. Although some literature such as fables provides direction for action, other literature describes suffering eloquently or recounts the experience from the perspective of the sufferer. Literature furnishes a view of suffering from inside the sufferer, providing vicarious experience and engaging the full humanity of the health-care professional. Study of literature can lead to compassionate care that complements the cognitive understanding of suffering and its attendant problems. For instance, many patients are unable to articulate their feelings and suffer silently. Literary works illuminate and promote greater understanding of the unexpressed dread, bewilderment, and meaninglessness of private suffering (Morris, 1996). Thus, prepared for an encounter that Dr. Edmund Pelligrino (1979) has described as ". . . the state of 'wounded humanity' of a person" (p. 45), health-care professionals ideally bring their knowledge, skills, and personal resources to a unique and irreplaceable suffering human being.

Literature provides a repertoire of possible answers to the questions, "What is suffering?" and "What is it like for patients?" enabling the health-care professional to more quickly and accurately determine the essence of a particular patient's suffering. Congruence between the patient's perception of his or her suffering and the caregiver's sense of that patient's suffering makes the patient feel less alone. It also furnishes positive feedback for the health-care professional that motivates continued efforts to understand, address, and relieve suffering. When the clinician fails to acknowledge and engage the patient's suffering, the patient may interpret silence as indifference. If inattention to suffering becomes a pattern of practice, health-care professionals are not only neglecting it but possibly blindly inflicting it (Moller, 1986–87). In the highest ideal of the professional calling, clinicians are obligated to see and hear suffering and to attempt to prevent and relieve it when they are in a position to do so. In the following pages, selected literary depictions of suffering illustrate the model of suffering and provide opportunity for the reader to experience temporarily what suffering is and to glimpse individual interpretations of isolation, hopelessness, vulnerability, and loss. Additional examples may be found in the Afterword.

ISOLATION

> No matter how surrounded by men, the sufferer is sometimes isolated, a hermit in the desert of his suffering.
> J.H. GRIFFITH (1970, P. 34)

In good health, we are normally part of a family, small groups, and the larger community; however, suffering distances patients from others and even from themselves. Conditions associated with illness and its treatment further isolate patients from their familiar routines. Although an illness may require the resources of a health-care facility, the process of institutionalization itself sometimes makes ongoing relationships with family and others difficult to sustain. In some cases, moreover, institutions tend to "take over" the illness; thereby, families feel excluded, and patients are encouraged to relinquish control (May, 1991). When patients encounter or are surrounded by health-care professionals who elect to distance themselves from suffering, the feeling of isolation is intensified.

Modern patients may share the aloneness that the ailing English poet John Donne, who lived from 1572 to 1631, expressed when he wrote, "As Sicknesse [sic] is the greatest misery, so the greatest misery of sicknesse [sic] is solitude . . .. Even the *Physician* dares scarse come" (Raspa, 1975, pp. 24–25). In extreme cases, sufferers who feel isolated may even regard themselves as having been banished and buried prematurely (May, 1991).

Some suffering persons experience not only a sense of separation from nurturing relationships but also a feeling of being detached from themselves. They may feel changed by a power beyond their control and believe that their identity has been altered (Mason, 1977). Griffith (1970) described this special kind of aloneness as "acting on two planes" (p. 27). For example, patients who experience unrelieved pain may have the feeling that they are *observing* their own pain. Other patients may be distressed by the difference between their former healthy state and their present symptomatic self that may seem unreal. Literature provides insights. In *The Death of Ivan Ilych* (1886/1971), Leo Tolstoy, who lived from 1828 to 1910, describes the private suffering of the central character, Ivan:

> Ivan Ilych saw that he was dying, and he was in continual despair. In the depth of his heart he knew he was dying, but not only was he not accustomed to the thought, he did not and could not grasp it (p. 44).

One recognizes the feeling of separation from the self and the consequent aloneness of Ivan through Tolstoy's description of his suffering. Ivan's lonely struggle to come to terms with the fact that he is dying of cancer is made difficult by the nature of the disease and the lie those who surround him sustain that he is not terminally ill.

Other sufferers, like Ivan, also dwell in a narrowed world because their suffering tends to fill their whole being. Alone with their suffering, nothing else seems to exist but their anguish. Other aspects of life fade as their focus on the suffering intensifies—they are unable to speak of little else or to speak at all. A patient's anguish may be exaggerated when he or she interprets symptoms to be destructive in themselves or to represent destruction of the body. In *Night*, published in 1960, Eli Wiesel writes poignantly of this intense focus when he struggled to survive starvation during his imprisonment as a teenager in a Nazi concentration camp. Wiesel wrote:

> I took little interest in anything except my daily plate of soup and my crust of stale bread. Bread, soup—these were my whole life. I was a body. Perhaps less than that even: a starved stomach. The stomach alone was aware of the passage of time (p. 50).

Thus sufferers wander unaccompanied in a solitary and frightening world in which they are separated by their conditions from normal relationships and perceptions of self and are left to dwell with suffering. Like the Ancient Mariner, they too feel:

> Alone, alone—all, all alone,
> Alone on a wide, wide sea!
> And never a saint took pity on
> My soul in agony
> (PART IV, LINES 232–235,
> COLERIDGE, 1797/1895, P. 57).

HOPELESSNESS

> I could lie down like a tired child
> And weep away the life of care
> Which I have borne and yet must bear.
> PERCY BYSSHE SHELLEY
> STANZAS WRITTEN IN *DEJECTION NEAR*
> *NAPLES* (BARNARD, 1944, P. 82,
> LINES 30–32)

In this excerpt, the reader readily senses the poet Shelley's (1792–1822) despair and his belief that his condition is unalterable. It is a feeling that many persons experience to some degree during illness. Hopelessness may be related to a current problem or condition or to the patient's inability to see beyond the present situation to other perspectives or sources of help (Farran, 1995). Patients who feel hopeless may be immobilized and unable to take action to change their situation or, in some cases, their behavior may be inappropriate (Farran, 1995).

Research suggests that hope and hopelessness do not exist on opposite ends of a continuum but as a dynamic state. For example, patients with poor prognoses may feel hopeless about recovering from their diseases, yet be hopeful that the symptoms will be well controlled and that they will remain comfortable because of the diligence of health-care professionals. Le Gresley (1991) confirmed this view with a qualitative study of burn patients. The investigator found that ". . . hope and hopeless are not mutually exclusive, and that hope is not the complete absence of hopelessness" (p. 180). This study alerts health- care professionals of the need to seek a desirable expectation with the patient, even in a critical situation that seems without resolution or cure.

Patients who feel hopeless differ from one another in their behavior because their responses are often shaped by prior experience with adversity. Some patients appear to be resigned and may be reticent about expressing their feelings. In *The Cancer Ward,* a novel about suffering and eventual freedom published in 1968, the author Solzhenitsyn (b. 1918) depicted dispassionate hopelessness. Early in the novel, Kostogotov, a patient, recounts his hopelessness during his illness:

> I was in agony for six months, and in the last month, I could no longer lie down nor sit nor stand without pain and I slept only a few minutes a day; I managed to think a few things out. That autumn I learned from my own example that a man can cross the threshold of death before his body is lifeless. Your blood may still be circulating, but—psychologically—you have gone through the whole preparation for death and endured death itself. You already see everything around you dispassionately, as from the grave (p. 37).

In contrast to Kostogotov's expression of his hopelessness, some suffering patients describe their sense of being out of control or caught up in chaos. They may relate their inability to identify alternatives or describe feeling overwhelmed. In the following excerpt, Ivan Ilych has been engulfed by hopelessness. The reader senses a tone of desperation as Ivan laments his suffering and impending death:

> . . . then he restrained himself no longer but wept like a child. He wept on account of his helplessness, his terrible loneliness, the cruelty of God, and the absence of God. "Why hast Thou done all this?" "Why hast Thou brought me here?" "Why, why dost Thou torment me so terribly?"
>
> (TOLSTOY, 1886/1971, P. 62).

In the end, Ivan's pitiful state is mitigated when he confronts and transcends his fear of death and finds hope beyond his illness.

VULNERABILITY AND LOSS

> Me miserable! Which way shall I fly
> Infinite wrath and infinite despair?
> Which way I fly is Hell; myself am Hell;
> And in the lowest deep, a lower deep
> Still threatening to devour me opens wide
> To which the Hell I suffer seems
> a heaven.

MILTON, 1665/1935
(BOOK 4, LINES 73–78, P. 81)

In this passage from the epic poem, *Paradise Lost,* John Milton (1608–1674) depicted the human feeling of vulnerability and loss. Completed about 1665, the poem's lines describe suffering in a manner that is familiar to the modern reader as all enveloping, relentless, and inescapable. As in the poem, vulnerability and loss coexist commonly in sufferers, although they can be distinguished intellectually. Patients who feel vulnerable believe that they are capable of being injured or experiencing greater injury, either physically or psychologically. When a loss has occurred, patients perceive that they lack something they expected to obtain or retain, and perhaps they fear vulnerability to greater loss. Patients may believe they have been damaged whether the loss is actual or perceived, and they may dread the prospect of greater harm.

Experienced clinicians are able to recall many situations in which patients have lived with both vulnerability and loss. For example, a patient with advanced congestive heart failure and unstable angina may experience the loss of gainful employment opportunities. This person may also feel vulnerable because he or she believes that susceptibility to greater disability and death will result from the pathology. According to Karl Jaspers (1969–71), vulnerability and the anticipation of death are critical to the definition of suffering. He wrote: ". . . [Suffering is] a restriction of existence, a partial destruction; behind all suffering looms the specter of death" (p. 202).

Patients typically feel some degree of vulnerability when unmistakable signs of disease appear or when a condition is diagnosed; however, they may be unable to articulate their feelings. This situation was captured and explicated by Albert Camus (1913–1960) in *The Plague (Le Peste)* (1948). The story described the spread of the bubonic plague in Oran, Algeria, in the 1940s. The work's political or philosophical themes are often the focus of literary study, but its depiction of anguished human beings as they confront suffering and death from a highly communicable disease is equally as imperative a focus. In the novel, the physician, Dr. Rieux, visits the ill daughter of Mme. Loret. Camus conveys the mother's vulnerability and sense of impending loss. On greeting the physician, Mme. Loret says, "I hope it is not the fever everyone is talking about." Then:

> Lifting the coverlet, he [Dr. Rieux] gazed in silence at the red blotches on the girl's thighs and stomach, the swollen ganglia. After one glance, the mother broke into shrill uncontrollable cries of grief. And every evening, mothers wailed thus, with distraught abstraction, as their eyes fell on those fatal stigmata on limbs and bellies; every evening hands gripped Rieux's arms . . . (p. 83).

Vulnerability and loss are often companions; in suffering, loss may either precede or follow vulnerability, and the situation may also be dynamic. Loss is related often to bodily dysfunction and the resultant changes in the character of the patient's existence. In a 1993 in-depth study of 57 chronically ill patients, for example, Charmaz learned that suffering was related to restrictions on patients' ability to control their lives, social isolation, and negative self-perceptions. The report of the study concluded, "The language of suffering these severely debilitated people spoke was the language of loss" (p. 91). The investigator asserted that the essential source of suffering was loss of the self.

In bereavement and death, a person's focus is predictably on loss, but isolation, hopelessness, and vulnerability are often involved as well. Recognition of the existence of these other dimensions requires attention to them as part of supporting those who are grieving and those who are dying. Centuries ago, the Christian theologian St. Augustine (354–430 CE) described his own suffering and grief about the death of a boyhood friend who did not survive a fever. In *Confessions* (c. 397/1912), St. Augustine first describes his aloneness and hopelessness:

> At the grief of this, my heart was utterly over clouded; and whatsoever I cast mine eyes upon, looked like death unto me. Mine own country was a very prison to me, and my father's house a wonderful unhappiness; and whatsoever I had communicated in with him, wanting him turned to my most cruel torture. Mine eyes roved about everywhere for him, but they met not with him
> (ST. AUGUSTINE, WATTS [WATTS, TRANS.], 1912, BOOK IV, CHAPTER IV, P. 161).

Then St. Augustine recalls his youthful sense of vulnerability and his loss of faith:

I became a great riddle to myself, and I often asked over my soul, why she was so sad, and why she afflicted me so sorely: but she knew not what to answer me. And if I said, "Put thy trust in God," very justly she did not obey me; . . .

(BOOK IV, CHAPTER IV, P. 161).

In these passages, St. Augustine not only mourns the loss of his friend, he also describes his inability to overcome the loss and find meaning. Because readers are moved by the expression of St. Augustine's suffering, they are able to empathize, momentarily, with what he feels and are thereby better able to understand what a patient or a patient's loved ones experience in similar circumstances. The reader is drawn into the feeling of loss of meaning and futility that may be the most enduring deprivation of all.

Meaning and Loss of Meaning

Suffering itself has no meaning. Humans, however, interpret all life circumstances, including illness, either by applying meaning or by discovering significance that seems to exist inherently (Blocker, 1974). Patients appear better able to bear suffering if meaning can be ascribed, because meaning relates their present powerlessness to an enduring and real belief that exists in spite of the suffering. Stable beliefs are a touchstone for decision making, even in chaos, and they may help patients to make choices, feel greater control, and view their distress in perspective. The notion that the disease treatment may provide useful medical information of benefit to others, that the sufferer may become stronger after recovery, or that God is present in the suffering are perspectives that can transform the suffering and the sufferer.

Meaninglessness, in contrast, may make the suffering nearly unbearable. In the following excerpts from *Night* (1960), the reader can perceive the agony of 15-year-old Elie Wiesel on his arrival at Birkenau, the reception center for Auschwitz. In the following passage, the reader senses his terror:

Never shall I forget that night, the first night in camp which has turned my life into one long night, seven times cursed and seven times sealed. Never shall I forget that smoke. Never shall I forget the little faces of the children whose bodies I saw turn into wreaths of smoke beneath a silent blue sky. Never shall I forget those flames which consumed my faith forever (p. 32).

Then, one glimpses the meaninglessness that this experience imposed upon him, as he continues:

Never shall I forget that nocturnal silence which deprived me, for all eternity, of the desire to live. Never shall I forget those moments which murdered my God and my soul and turned dreams to dust. Never shall I forget these things even if I am condemned to live as long as God Himself. Never. (p. 32).

Although the Auschwitz imprisonment robbed him of meaning, Elie Wiesel found a new life purpose after his release by recounting the horrors inflicted by the Nazis on the Jews and others and by reporting the collective and individual suffering of these peoples during the Holocaust or Shoah.

Hearing Patients Express Suffering

What inundates a traumatized life is, really, at once overwhelming, void of meaning, and unsayable. That is what people in pain are telling us, if only we will hear.

A. EGENDORF (1995, P. 20)

In the early section of this chapter, the impediments to perceiving suffering were identified to encourage clinicians to see suffering that exists. Then the reader was invited to expand the cognitive understanding of the model of suffering by examining the perspectives of selected disciplines and by scrutinizing individual suffering through the lens of literature. Now it is important to examine how to listen to what initially may be difficult for the patient to express and to begin to then determine its significance.

Patients suffer when they perceive that an event or a force has changed their lives adversely or that a desired situation will not occur. Generally suffering related to illness is an ongoing state that may vary in content and intensity from day to day or even from hour to hour. In addition, the sources or meaning of suffering may evolve or be different during the course of an illness. This fluidity makes a single, definitive evaluation of or response to suffering seemingly impossible.

When patients are able to express their distress, they may do so in different ways. They may seem anguished, indifferent, uncooperative, or angry. Some persons even use suffering to manipulate or cause distress in others. Just as health-care professionals need to see and become sensitive to suffering, so too they must learn to perceive suffering in words and in behavior beyond the language of the patient who is overwhelmed.

PRESENTATION OF SUFFERING

Reich (1989) has written that suffering may be either mute or expressive. In mute suffering, words cannot be used to describe emotion. The patient may scream, be silent, or weep. Mme. Loret's cry in the excerpt from *The Plague,* quoted previously, is an example of her mute suffering when she saw the unmistakable signs of the plague on her daughter's body and realized that her child would die of the disease in a short time. Health-care professionals need to understand that patients who are mute may not be able to comprehend what is being said to them or perhaps may be able to hear only simple sentences such as, "I'm sorry that this has happened to you" or "How can I make you more comfortable?" Learned professional responses such as, "Tell me how you feel.," are *not* appropriate in such situations. Being present and sharing the experience with the sufferer is more helpful.

Responses to expressive suffering, articulated through language, require a more active role for the clinician. Although some patients withdraw for a prolonged period because they seek to avoid their anguish or are attempting to process it, most eventually represent their suffering in words. As identified by Reich (1989), expressive suffering has three phases: lament, narration of the story, and discovery of a new meaning.

Lament

Each phase requires a different response. The word *lament* means to express deep sorrow and is not commonly heard in health-care facilities. Clinicians sometimes describe those patients who lament as "complainers" and may view them as weak, whining persons. Such patients may even be labeled as troublesome or are avoided. In labeling, health-care providers are failing to appreciate that these patients are articulating their suffering in the only way they can and need a forbearing and caring person to listen.

Historically, lamenting, particularly in some cultures, has been an accepted behavior and often has been part of the healing process wherein sufferers have found hope and confidence that a better future awaits them. An ancient example may be found in the *Old Testament* book of *Lamentations*. The first 64 verses describe starvation, death, and other suffering that occurred when Jerusalem was vanquished in 586 BCE. Then the account continues with these words of transcendency:

> Yet hope returns when I
> remember one thing:
> The Lord's unfailing love and
> Mercy still continue,
> Fresh as the morning, as

sure as the sunrise.
The Lord is all I have, and
in Him I put my hope (*Lamentations 3*, 22–24).

Today's patients are often given neither permission nor opportunity to lament. During ever shorter hospital stays, acutely ill patients are frequently pressured to behave as if they have recovered. Immediately following a mastectomy, or even before surgery, for example, some patients are exhorted to be "cancer survivors." When such patients are not in a caring context or known as individuals, when the caregiver lacks expertise to predict outcomes, or when the notion of "being a survivor" is thrust on them prematurely, it can *cause* suffering. Rather than engendering hope, even a well-intended clinician may isolate the patient by imposing a perspective or a meaning that is not congruent with the patient's readiness to embrace it. Insensitivity to the life-changing impact of cancer surgery is evident when the health-care professional fails to take into account that the woman needs time to mourn her lost body part, to be comforted by religion, and/or to discover a personal meaning related to what is at stake for her. It is far easier and more comfortable for the clinician to simply exhort a patient to "be a survivor" than to share her anguish until she is ready to embrace that view.

Narrative

Although mute suffering may be missed, and laments may be unheard as cries for caring, health-care professionals are more frequently attuned to patients' articulated struggles to resolve the trauma. Unfortunately, health-care professionals in acute-care settings infrequently see this time of restoration because of limited hospital stays.

While the patient's story in the lament may seem unorganized or even chaotic, the narrative begins to take form, and patients may engage the caregiver in a dialogue as they attempt to create a more hopeful story (Reich, 1989). Expressions of self-blame may begin to evolve; for example, a cancer patient might say, "I should not have postponed my mammogram." In this stage, the clinician may gently affirm the patient with, "Yes, go on." or offer more positive support with a statement such as, "Now you have a good treatment plan." In time, some patients see beyond the traumatic event without becoming overwhelmed. The health-care professional may support the change in perception with clarification and validation and some tentative interpretative statements such as, "You seem to be saying that you are viewing your condition more hopefully."

Significance

Just as suffering is experienced uniquely, so too the manner in which patients find significance in their suffering is singular. Clues as to how meaning is constructed may be determined by listening to patients. For example, does the patient ascribe blame for the suffering or view the suffering as avoidable or predetermined or attributable to natural causes? Pre-existing religious or philosophical beliefs associated with such questions may be rejected, questioned, modified, or reaffirmed by the patient. Optimally, the view that emerges will enable the patient to move toward acceptance or a more personally satisfying view of his situation. For instance, parents who blame themselves for lack of diligence resulting in the injury of a child may be comforted by accepting that the injury resulted from an unforeseen random happening, modifying their view that the world is predictable. Moreover, knowing that other devoted, vigilant parents have experienced similar events may ultimately alleviate some of their suffering by modifying their sense of guilt and isolation.

Walking through suffering with another person requires sensitivity, competence, courage, and intention to encounter expressed and unexpressed suffering. Yet some tragedy seems not to be amenable to relief. We cannot succeed always, but we cannot profess to be healers if we fail to be sensitive to suffering, prevent unnecessary suffering, and be present to assist patients to bear suffering. When we fail to act, we are morally responsible for the harm caused by the inaction (James, 1982). Although some clinicians do avoid or even flee from suffering, encountering patients' suffering is more than an obligation, according to David Gregory (1994) who has observed that "Offering a privilege of the highest magnitude, patients choose those who will journey through suffering with them" (p. 22).

SUMMARY _____

Health-care professionals may neglect the suffering of their patients because they are inexperienced or lacking in relevant knowledge about the nature of suffering. They may believe that science will "cure" suffering, suffering can be relieved quickly and fully, or relief requires only clinical activity without investment of the self. Clinicians find in the behavioral and social sciences, theories and strategies that clarify and contribute to the resolution of certain emotional and situational problems of the suffering person. Religion and philosophy furnish contextual understandings of suffering. Literature enables health-care professionals to see suffering by experiencing it vicariously and also by developing a repertoire of examples of how human beings experience and express suffering. Listening for patients' expressions of suffering requires intention, an understanding of how suffering may be represented, sensitivity and skill in framing an appropriate response, or the wisdom just to be empathically present and silent. The health-care professional must be aware also of how the patient interprets the suffering. Meaning and significance will be considered in the next chapter.

PRECEPT FOR PRACTICE

It is incumbent on health-care professionals to make a conscious effort to see, hear, and encounter hurt because knowledge of the physical disorder alone may furnish limited guidance.

REFERENCES

Barnard, E. (Ed.). (1944). *Shelley: Selected poems, essays and letters.* New York: The Odyssey.

Blocker, H. (1974). *The Meaning of Meaninglessness.* The Hague: Martinuis Nijhoff.

Camus, A. (1948). *The Plague.* New York: Modern Library.

Charmaz, K. (1993). Loss of self: A fundamental form of suffering in the chronically ill. *Sociology of Health and Illness, 5*(2), 168–95.

Coleridge, S. (1904). *The rime of the ancient mariner.* New York: American Book Company.

Egendorf, A. (1995). Hearing people through their pain. *Journal of Traumatic Stress, 8*(1), 5–28.

Eliot, G. (1859/1917). *Adam Bede.* Chicago: Charles Scribner's Sons.

Farran, C., et al. (1995). *Hope and hopelessness: Critical clinical constructs.* Thousand Oaks, Calif.: Sage Publications.

Fordyce, Wilbert E. (1988). Pain and suffering: A reappraisal. *American Psychologist, 43,* 276–83.

Good News Bible (1992). New York: American Bible Society.

Gregory, D. (1994). The myth of control: Suffering in palliative care. *Journal of Palliative Care, 10*(2), 18–22.

Griffith, J.H. (1970). The terrain of physical pain. In A. Paton, et al. (Eds.), *Creative suffering: The ripple of hope* (pp. 25–37). Philadelphia: The Pilgrim Press; and Kansas City, MO: The National Catholic Reporter.

James, S. (1982). The duty to relieve suffering. *Ethics, 93,* 4–21.

Jaspers, K. (1969–1971). *Philosophy,* Volume 2. (E.B. Ashton, trans.). Chicago: University of Chicago Press.

Le Gresley, A. (1991). Hopelessness. In *NANDA, classification of nursing diagnoses. Proceedings of the Ninth Conference,* Philadelphia: J.B. Lippincott.

Liegner, L.M. (1986–87). Suffering. *Loss, Grief and Care, 1,* 93–96.

Mason, D. (1977). Some abstract, yet critical thoughts about suffering. *Dialogue, 16,* 91–100.

May, W. (1991). *The patient's ordeal.* Bloomington, Ind.: Indiana University Press.

Milton, J. (1665/1935). *Paradise lost.* New York: The Odyssey Press.

Moller, D.W. (1986–87). On the value of suffering in the shadow of death. *Loss, Grief and Care, 1,* 127–36.

Morris, D. (1996). About suffering: Voice, genre, and moral community. *Daedalus, 125*(1), 23–45.

Pelligrino, E. (1979). Toward a reconstruction of medical morality: The primacy of the act of profession and the fact of illness. *The Journal of Medicine and Philosophy, 4*(1), 32–56.

Raspa, A. (Ed.). (1975). *John Donne: Devotions on emergent occasions.* Montreal: McGill-Queens University Press.

Rawlinson, M. (1986). The sense of suffering. *Journal of Medicine and Philosophy, 11,* 39–62.

Reich, W.T. (1989). Speaking of suffering: A moral account of compassion. *Soundings, 72,* 83–108.

Saint Augustine (c. 397–401/1912). *Confessions,* Volume 1. (W. Watts, trans.). London: William Heinemann.

Sarason, S. (1985). *Caring and compassion in clinical practice.* San Francisco: Jossey-Bass.

Solzhenitsyn, A. (1968). *The cancer ward.* (R. Frank, Trans.). New York: The Dial Press.

Tolstoy, L. (1886/1971). The death of Ivan Ilych. In L. Maude & A. Maude (trans.), *The death of Ivan Ilych and other stories* (pp. 1–73) New York: Oxford University Press.

Wiesel, E. (1960). *Night.* New York: Bantam Books.

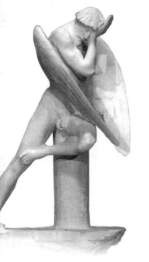

Chapter 4

How Is Significance Found in Suffering?

> Every one of us, in the time of suffering, has opportunity to bear witness to the unseen things through the seen quality of his demeanor.
>
> H.W. ROBINSON (1939, P. 214)

"How can I endure this suffering?" "What will be the outcome of my illness?" and "What is to become of me?" are common questions that signal spiritual or existential distress. These queries are quests for meaning in suffering, and it is important for clinicians to understand whether the patient's concerns are of a religious or spiritual nature.

Patients, just like persons who are healthy, must seek, discover, and integrate significance and purpose into their lives. And like people everywhere, patients are at different stages of imbuing their experience with meaning. For some patients, suffering brings a sense that they have encountered a malevolent power greater than themselves (Steeves & Kahn, 1997). For example, a patient diagnosed with an inoperable tumor may define it as evil and be terrified to realize that the pathology will render him or her helpless and result in death. But other patients find meaning in their suffering by relating to God, to a Supreme Being, or to an Ultimate Reality. Still other patients exist in an "existential vacuum" (Starck & McGovern, 1992, p. 27) wherein the illness is seemingly without meaning. They may feel fearful and powerless because the illness and suffering seem out of control, and they are consequently without consolation.

Because the significance a patient ascribes to suffering can influence his or her experience either positively or negatively, health-care professionals need to be sensitive to the meaning that exists beyond the specifics of the patient's condition. When the meaning detected is negative and adds to the patient's distress, counseling, particularly spiritual counseling, may be in order. It may help also when patients express a sense of meaninglessness because sometimes the meaning of suffering just awaits discovery.

Although it is tempting for health-care professionals to offer patients philosophical or religious perspectives, their intentions can sometimes be insensitive. When a point of view has not been invited by the patient, or is incongruent with his or her views, it may make the patient feel even less understood and alone, thereby adding to the suffering. However, when clinicians assist patients to identify a meaning that helps patients to endure their suffering, patients can often find sustenance.

The purpose of this chapter is to help clinicians develop an awareness of the significance that patients may ascribe to illness and suffering and show how that understanding can help to ameliorate suffering. Broad viewpoints are discussed as well as precepts of the four dominant religions in the United States. These perspectives serve to sensitize health-care professionals to selected transcendent sources of strength or the characteristics that Larry Dossey (1989) has called "nonlocal—the mind—that is infinite in space and time . . . (p. 79).

Seeking Purpose and Meaning

Any patient is free to select a health-care professional, other type of caregiver, or clergy member to engage in philosophical, spiritual, or religious conversations. In these situations, the patient's choice must be honored. Although the selected caregiver may feel inadequate, seeking consultation while respecting confidentiality may help both patient and caregiver. Rector Paul Chidwick (1988) suggests a sensitive approach, based on his hospice experience, to assist patients searching for meaning in their illness. He writes:

> Anyone who is engaged in the search for life's meaning will appreciate pastoral help. The word *pastoral* has strong associations with the concept of shepherding. And it is the work of a shepherd gently to guide people in their spiritual journeys, not to drag them through a prescribed route (p. 87).

Religion, narrowly defined, encompasses the beliefs and practices of those who profess a specific faith. By being aware of the basic religious beliefs of patients in their community, health-care professionals can better understand how patients may explain suffering and what consolation their faith may offer. *Salvation, sin,* and *grace* are examples of terms identified by Doyle (1992) that alert a caregiver to a patient who may be imbuing suffering with a religious meaning. The caregiver should refer these patients to a clergy member or other religious resources for appropriate support.

While spirituality may include religious beliefs, it is broader and relates to the basic holistic concerns of being human, according to Doyle. The spirit (or soul) connotes matters that are more than physical, material, or worldly such as hopelessness, vulnerability, anger, and fear of death (Speck, 1988). Marsilio Ficino, writing in the 15th century, described *spirit* or *soul* as a bridge between mind and body. As quoted in *Care of the Soul,* he observes:

> The mind . . . tends to go off on its own so that it seems to have no relevance to the physical world. At the same time, the materialistic life can be so absorbing that we get caught up in it and forget about spirituality. What we need is soul, in the middle, holding together mind and body, . . . (Moore, 1992, pp. xiii–xiv).

Modern health-care professionals may be insensitive to the spiritual dimension of care. More commonly they are uncomfortable when patients express their spirituality by asking existential questions. Accustomed to curing through technology, such health-care professionals wrongly feel that they are doing little or nothing if they simply listen when patients describe their suffering and their attempts to make sense of it. Listening and mutually seeking an interpretation of the suffering can guide the patient in the healing quest for meaning that transcends the here and now. Even in situations in which the patient and the clinician may literally speak different languages, the sufferer may benefit by the attentiveness and presence of a sensitive caregiver rather than through advanced technology. Gilje (1992) describes presence as not only "being there" physically (or on call) but also "being with" a patient emotionally and spiritually (pp. 56–57). Presence requires that the clinician acknowledge patients' humanity, individuality, and suffering, and that interactions be open and without intent to manipulate. Clinicians may simply convey a willingness to accompany patients as they bear their suffering, even when those patients may be unlovable strangers. Some kinds of suffering cannot be cured or fixed quickly, if at all. Relieving suffering is a process, and the outcome is never certain. A patient's crushed arm may be repaired and the wound healed; however, the patient may perceive himself or herself as a "useless cripple" and suffer for months or for all of life although the residual physical damage may be minimal. Indeed, some kinds of suffering are so tragic for patients that they never experience relief. Sometimes the suffering remains in the mind or in the body without the spirit to hold them together and make the patient whole.

Theistic and Nontheistic Views

Sensitivity to suffering, willingness to acknowledge it, awareness of the spiritual and religious dimensions of living, and appreciation that suffering may be transformed are minimal expectations of those who care for the ill. Clinicians who wish to become more competent, however, seek greater understanding of common perspectives that may construct how patients both experience and articulate suffering, often with a sense of relatedness to something greater than themselves. Comforting patients and shepherding them in their search for meaning or allowing them to seek their own meaning involves the ability to differentiate nontheistic from theistic ideologies.

Patients with a theistic perspective believe in the existence of God (monotheism) or gods (pantheism, polytheism). In contrast, atheists are those ". . . without a belief in God, not necessarily someone who believes that God does not exist" (Martin, 1990, p. 463), whereas the agnostic ". . . neither believes nor disbelieves that God exists" (p. 466). The theistic views discussed in this chapter (Judaism, Christianity, and Islam) regard God as a divine ruler who is involved in the affairs of humans. Buddhism exemplifies a nontheistic perspective that lacks a transcendent God and stresses personal responsibility for self-development and spiritual growth. Familiarity with these broad ideologies may enable clinicians to discern, in a general way, how patients' views may shape their suffering and imbue it with meaning. Some patients, however, focus entirely on the here and now and lack a coherent ideology for interpreting their suffering (Nouwen, 1972).

THEISTIC VIEWS

Perspectives that seek meaning for suffering in supernatural beliefs that ascribe happenings to a divine being or force (Watson, 1986–87) are described as *theistic*. Theists believe typically that God is both personal and responsive to human beings. According to Gibbs (1988), there are alternative views within theistic beliefs. The first is the "theistic-sovereign" (pp. 22–24) view, which emphasizes that God controls the world. Patients with this theological view may regard their illness and suffering as divine punishment or may look on it as a test of faith and then hope for divine intervention and deliverance.

When patients with theistic-sovereign beliefs tell a caregiver that God is punishing them with illness for their sins, it is neither appropriate nor comforting to the patient to reply, "You seem like such a good person. You could not have done anything that wrong." However well intended, this reply amounts to rejection of the manner in which the patient has made sense of his suffering. The patient's interpretation of the clinician's statement is: "You don't understand what I believe," "You don't care about my experience and my faith," and "You can't help me with my suffering." A better response by the clinician would be, "It must be distressing to feel as you do. Would it be helpful to discuss your feelings with someone—perhaps a chaplain?" In this reply, the suffering is acknowledged, and the theistic-sovereign views are honored, making the patient feel understood. Additionally, a referral is offered to put the patient into contact with a qualified person who can deal with those personal and specific religious issues that contribute to the patient's perceptions. Perhaps healing rituals and absolution can be offered as well.

The other theistic view Gibbs identified is the "theistic-consoling" (pp. 24–26) view. This view stresses the presence of God's love in difficult and tragic situations. References by patients to God's understanding of suffering, God's ability to comfort the sufferer, and the hope of union with a loving God after death often distinguish patients with theistic-consoling beliefs. Such patients may benefit from clinicians who affirm God's love and care in life, tragedy, and suffering.

NONTHEISTIC VIEWS

Nontheistic ideas do not ascribe suffering to supernatural forces. Buddhism does not embrace a deity who intervenes in human affairs. Buddhists seek to live amidst suffering and use their own initiative to find an ultimate state—*Nirvana.* Likewise, secular humanists emphasize that people can manage their own lives without reference to God as a personal being or controller of the universe. Humanists are concerned primarily with what is distinctively human, such as the ability to reason, rather than with ultimate purpose and absolute moral standards (Lamont, 1949). They hold that humans are responsible for what they become (McDowell & Stewart, 1989). Some humanists do not exclude God entirely but place relatively less emphasis on God than do those with theistic views (p. 459).

Thus, sensitive caregivers understand that suffering is related to patients' spiritual states. Whether spirituality is understood to include philosophy and the higher qualities of the mind, or whether it involves the soul and is expressed through religion, this noncorporeal entity is an important means of determining the source of suffering and identifying some resources for relieving it.

Spirituality is not limited by the current state of the mind or body. Dossey (1989) defined this state as "local and isolated" (p. 248). Rather, spirituality involves "nonlocal being," which is a way of experiencing suffering by seeking something of transcendent value, described by Dossey (1989) in *Recovering the Soul.* In the following excerpt, he summarizes the potential of nonlocal being to relieve suffering:

> Participation in nonlocal being is nothing less than *spiritual morphine:* it reduces pain and suffering. But unlike a medication, it does not last only until the "injection" wears off, leaving one to face more pain and anguish. The analgesia of nonlocal being is curative, not palliative, for it eliminates the root and source of suffering: the isolated person, the self who is trapped in time and finite space, drifting toward destruction (p. 236).

Four Views of Suffering and Its Significance

As discussed earlier, feelings of hopelessness, loneliness, vulnerability, loss, and fear indicate that a patient is suffering and may be spiritually searching. In the broadest sense, religion can be equated with spirituality. As defined in the *Encyclopedia Americana, 1996,* religion is:

> . . . the pattern of belief and practice through which men communicate with or hope to gain experience of that which lies beyond the world of their ordinary experience. Typically, it focuses on an ultimate or absolute, thought of by some believers as God (p. 359).

Substantial numbers of persons in the United States participate in or state a preference for four major religions: Christianity (131,084,000 persons), Judaism (3,137,000 persons), Islam (527,000 persons), and Buddhism (401,000 persons) (*Statistical Abstracts of the United States, 1998,* pp. 71–72). In various regions of the United States, many patients will be part of these religious groups or influenced by these religious beliefs; therefore, some discourse follows about the basic tenets of each religion, its views of suffering, and its consolations. The information is offered as a guide to health-care professionals when they attend to patients who seek to interpret and find meaning for their suffering. It is important to remember, however, that some beliefs and practices of a religion may vary from culture to culture and over time. Even more significant is the caution that the beliefs of subgroups or individuals may vary from orthodox views accepted by the respective religions.

Each religion to be discussed, in order of historical development, provides humans with what Edward Jurji (1958) described as an enduring Ultimate Reality. He noted that for Jews, the central belief is that God is revealed in history and the scriptures. God is a transcendent mystery and is beyond present events and tragedy. The idea of God for Christians emphasizes that God is the Loving Redeemer and that humans can be saved from sin and achieve salvation through the death and resurrection of Jesus. Judgment and the absolute power of God (Allah) in all aspects of life is the center of Islamic belief. For the Buddhists, the Ultimate Reality is that mental and spiritual enlightenment enables human beings to attain spiritual release (Nirvana).

JUDAISM

Basic Beliefs

Judaism began with the Jewish patriarchs (Abraham, Isaac, and Jacob) about 4000 years ago and has as its central belief the concept of one God (YHWH). This belief is captured in the solemn prayer (the Sh'ma), "Hear, O Israel, our God Adonai is One" (Robinson, 2000, p. 33). Within Judaism, God is found in all creation. God's will, mystery, and commandments are revealed in history. This belief is affirmed in the last line of a prayer, "Yet to every generation hast thou revealed a portion of the mystery of thy Being" (Glatzer, 1974, p. 25). God's will for human beings, especially the Jews, is conveyed in the *Torah* (the Five Books of Moses), which is a record of authoritative teaching and divine revelation (de Lang, 1986). In Judaism, God and Man are bound together by a covenant (*brit*) in which humans who faithfully obey God will be protected by Him (Eisen, 1987). But Judaism also affirms that those who fail to obey God will be punished.

Although the foregoing beliefs are central to Judaism, there is considerable variety in the religion. It is not dogmatic in requiring all believers to accept all tenets. Instead, beliefs flow from historical experience (de Lange, 1986). Central to that experience is the sense of community through which an individual Jew is understood to be part of the Jewish people and nation. The importance of this sense of community is illuminated by the author who writes:

> To be a Jew means first and foremost to belong to a group, the
> Jewish people, and the religious beliefs are secondary, in a sense, to
> this corporate allegiance . . .. Indeed there are many people in the
> world who consider themselves to be loyal Jews in every respect and
> who would deny that they have any religion at all (pp. 4–5).

When clinicians encounter patients who are described on the
medical record as "Jewish," it is necessary to understand, according to
de Lange, that patients may define themselves as *secular* Jews
(nonreligious), or they may accept and participate in the religious
dimension of Judaism. Among those who are religious, moreover,
there are differences in perspective concerning traditional beliefs and
practices. *Traditionalism,* usually associated with small immigrant
groups in the West, is characterized by attempts to maintain historical
practices and beliefs and exclude modern thinking from Jewish life.
Modern movements, including orthodoxy, conservatism, and reform,
bring tradition into greater accord with modern life, but, "In their very
different ways they all profess the belief in a single, beneficent God
and in the authority of scripture, and they all maintain the institutions
of the synagogue and the rabbinate" (de Lange, 2000, p. 79).

In spite of these differences, clinicians need to be sensitive to the
importance of history, tradition, family, and community to their
Jewish patients. For example, traditional Jews are bound by historical
dietary laws (Kashrut) that need to be taken into consideration in
planning their care. These laws require that food be prepared in a
particular way (Kosher) and that some food be forbidden—such as
pork or fish without scales and fins (de Lange, p. 82). If such food is
presented to an ill person and not eaten, it may be because of religious
belief, not appetite or health state.

Suffering in Judaism

Like people of other traditions, Jews have sought to understand why
evil—including suffering—occurs. Suffering is thought to come about
through one's own actions, by the actions of others, or by virtue of the
fact that we have a body (Bowker, 1970). Suffering may be regarded as
a punishment for human actions that are displeasing to God.
Deuteronomy 3:15, for example, makes clear that evil things will
happen to those who do not keep God's laws. Included are crop and
weather disasters, property loss, agricultural failures, and political
upheaval. Certain illnesses are mentioned specifically as punishment:
epidemics of infectious diseases, boils, sores, itches without cure, loss
of mind, blindness, confusion, and incurable disease (*Deuteronomy*
28:16–68).

Patients who view suffering as punishment may feel more accepted if clinicians understand that they may regard suffering as a consequence of behavior; therefore, the appropriate course of action is for sufferers who are Jews to examine their actions, make amends, and repent (Fox, 1987). For example, a patient whose behavior has caused alienation from his parents may strive to make contact with them and heal the relationship. In this way, forgiveness and reunification with that which is divine may be achieved.

Another explanation for suffering in Judaism is that it is a test of faith. The *Old Testament* described the belief that God is ultimately just. For Job, who faced many trials, this belief was fulfilled—"The Lord blessed the last part of Job's life even more than he had blessed the first" (*Job* 42:12). Such perseverance and faith during suffering is described in the following 1492 prayer of a Jewish exile from Spain who had witnessed the death of his wife and two children:

> Lord of the universe,
> You are doing much to make me desert my faith.
> But I assure you that—even against the will of the dwellers in
>   heaven—a Jew I am and a Jew I shall remain
> and neither the sufferings that you have brought upon me nor that
>   which you will yet bring upon me will be of any avail (Glatzer,
> 1974, p. 74).

Persons who suffer loss without consolation are advised to, "Hold life with open arms" (Singer, 1989, p. 53), which means understanding that life's relationships and events are temporary, whereas God is eternal. These patients may be comforted by the idea that reverent persons can perceive that something greater than their present situation exists (Kushner, 1981) and that something may be learned from the experience of suffering (Hartman, 1978).

Among Jews, an additional explanation of suffering is that God allows suffering to occur although its ultimate purpose may not be understood. For some religious persons, this view is the essence of the *Book of Job.* The mystery of God's care is that Job suffered, but he did not sin. According to Rabbi Kushner (1981), "God does not send sickness or disease, accident or tragedy. Such things happen for reasons of human cruelty or foolishness or the laws of nature" (p. 94). When anguish does occur, however, patients may be comforted by the belief that suffering is finite in terms of eternity and that injustice will be compensated in the eternal purposes of God (Schlesinger, 1989, pp. 22–41). According to Schlesinger, some patients may take comfort also in seeing that even very distressing situations may have good aspects, such as the caring and compassionate acts of others, that in some cases, are even virtuous. For the Jew, the greatest consolation is that God, who is omnipotent and has revealed Himself in all times and in all places, can be *trusted* when suffering exists.

BUDDHISM

Buddhism was established in India about 2500 years ago (McDowell & Stewart, 1989). The founder was Siddhartha Gautama, the son of a wealthy ruler, who enjoyed a life of privilege in his early years. He was protected from natural and human tragedies and suffering. After leaving his father's palace, Siddhartha encountered an old person, a sick person, and a funeral procession that challenged his pleasure-oriented view of life. Disillusioned, he began a quest for meaning and wisdom that he ultimately achieved through extended meditation during which he reached the highest spiritual state. He spent the remainder of his life further developing his spiritual insights and teaching. As a consequence of the truths he discovered and shared, he became known as the Buddha—that is, the Enlightened One. The first of his Noble Truths was that life intrinsically involves suffering (Varadhammo, 1996). All human beings suffer pain and loss and eventually die. Job and Jesus also exemplified this Noble Truth of Buddhism.

Although Buddhism was well-established in India and the East, it was little known in Europe until the Crusaders and other European travelers visited areas where Buddhism was practiced. In the West, a serious study of Buddhism did not begin until written materials became available to scholars about 1800 CE (Robinson & Johnson, 1982). Currently, in the United States, most Buddhists are immigrants from southeast Asia (for example, Vietnam) and east Asia (China, Japan, and Korea), and their descendants (Bracken, personal communication, March, 2001); however, Caucasian Buddhists are growing in number because of influence by Buddhist teaching and missionary efforts (McDowell, 1989). Buddhism's spiritual emphasis is especially attractive to some persons who are discontent with secularism in modern life.

Basic Ideas

Buddhism may be regarded both as a philosophy of life and a religion; it is nontheistic (Kitagawa, 1989). Truth is *not* revealed by a supernatural being; it is discovered in experience and in the analysis of human self-awareness via mental discipline and meditation. For persons oriented to western thinking and its theistic religions and systems of dogma, Buddhism requires an openness to the idea that it is a way of life in which humans must find their own meaning and path to happiness through spiritual discipline. According to Hajime Nakamurr (Dumoulin, 1976), this admonition was made explicit by the Buddha in his last sermon:

> Be a lamp to yourself. Be a refuge to yourself. Betake yourself to no external refuge. Hold fast as a refuge to the truth. Don't look for a refuge to anyone besides yourself (p. 11).

Buddhism teaches that through spiritual discipline, humans can progress to the highest spiritual state, which is ". . . without pain, distress or sorrow." This state is known as *Nirvana* (Masutani, 1967), described as ". . . the Final and Ultimate Realization of the Spiritual Life" (Varadhammo, 1996, p. 17). It is achieved after multiple cycles of birth, death, and rebirth (Bareau, 1979). The nature of the rebirth will be pleasurable if the intentions and actions of a prior life were moral. Actions and intentions that violated moral rules lead to an unpleasant rebirth (Spiro, 1970). The consequence of moral acts is referred to as *karma*.

Suffering in Buddhism

Although suffering is an important consideration in some religions, it is absolutely central in Buddhism. Buddhists affirm that one must know what suffering is, what its cause is, and how it is extinguished— and how a state of no suffering is achieved. These insights of the Buddha are known as the *Four Noble Truths* (Varadhammo, 1996, pp. 99–128). Buddha defined suffering more broadly than is typical in western thinking as recorded by Masutani (1967):

> Now this, bhikkus [monks], is the noble truth of suffering: birth is suffering, sickness is suffering, death is suffering, sorrow, lamentation, dejection, and despair are suffering. Contact with unpleasant things is suffering, separation from the pleasing is suffering, not getting what one wishes is suffering (p. 14).

The patient who is a Buddhist, therefore, does not regard suffering to be imposed by a supernatural being (Birnbaum, 1979). Rather, suffering exists and has understandable natural causes (Bowker, 1970). Buddhism affirms *karma* as the universal law of cause and effect. Causes are natural and produce illness or injury that may be treated by scientific medicine and related mental and spiritual therapies.

According to Bowker, suffering and illness may also be the consequence of one's negative acts in another life (Law of Karma) or may become a source of spiritual development. Illness and suffering are related to the failure to appreciate that everything is impermanent and to the inability to manage craving or desire. In the Buddhist view, all things are temporary and changing; for example, good health is not permanent, and relationships may be altered or lost. This fact must be accepted. Craving what one lacks, fearing losing what one possesses, or failing to accept impermanence may cause spiritual illness.

Accordingly, Buddhist patients especially need a holistic approach to care that not only affirms the distress caused by the disease, but also acknowledges the patients' attempts to overcome suffering arising from impermanence in other aspects of life that accompanies the illness. Buddhism supports the perspective of many health-care professionals that understanding the relationship of body, mind, and spirit is essential to defining and healing illness.

Consolation

Buddhism does not concentrate on the purpose of suffering as do some other religions. Suffering, a universal condition, is an ever-present reality. The Buddhist confronts suffering directly and attempts to understand and overcome it. Mental discipline, analysis, and meditation are practiced by Buddhists. These skills may enable Buddhist patients to accept and overcome their situations through self-reliance.

Certain precepts may be especially comforting to those who suffer, such as the belief that death is a part of an ongoing process and is not to be dreaded because it is followed by rebirth and perhaps an ultimate spiritual state. Thus, the dead are missed but not mourned (Kitagawa, 1989, p. 30). The Buddhist who accepts the teaching that nothing is permanent, including the self, may be able to depersonalize bodily changes brought about by disease. Finally, the goal of detachment can be achieved by Buddhists via mental discipline and meditation that lead to insight. In this state, neither self nor suffering is perceived as real (Cooper, 1989). Quoting from *Dialogues of the Buddha* (Pt. II, p. 327) Spiro (1970) summarizes:

> [Meditation is] . . . the one and only path, Bhikkhus, leading to the purification of beings, to passing far beyond grief and lamentation, to the dying out of ill and misery . . . to the realization of Nirvana . . . (p. 53).

Clinicians can be helpful to Buddhist patients in the specific ways suggested by the precepts noted previously. These include understanding the explanations for illness and suffering, providing holistic care, demonstrating compassion that affirms universally shared suffering, and providing opportunities for meditation. More important, those clinicians whose experience has been in the western tradition need to become sensitive to and knowledgeable about the different world view of the Buddhist. Essentially, Buddhism is world renouncing and regards attachment to the world as a cause of suffering and an obstacle to spiritual maturation. Detachment from others, objects, and self is sought as a path to Nirvana, self-purification, and general well-being (Spiro, 1970). In the ultimate state of Nirvana, one transcends temporary imperfection, and suffering ceases. This destiny or possibility offers comfort to the Buddhist as he or she faces this life and its events, including suffering, because Nirvana ". . . depicts the Highest Wisdom attainable by Mankind. Above all, it is the final and Ultimate Realization of the Spiritual Life" (Varadhammo, 1996, p. 17).

CHRISTIANITY

Christianity grew out of the life experience and teachings of Jesus of Nazareth in Palestine about 2000 years ago (Bainton, 1964). As a Jewish reformist rabbi, Jesus incorporated traditional Jewish beliefs in his teaching, the purpose of which was to call the Jews back to God. He also modified the Law of Moses and reformulated it to include love of God and loving concern for neighbors without prior conditions (*agape*). In addition, Jesus also taught of the coming of God's kingdom on earth. These ideas not only attracted followers, but also created tension within Judaism, according to the author. Because Jesus was hailed by some of his followers as *Messiah* (Deliverer of the Jews), his teachings challenged the Roman government that occupied Palestine at that time. Jesus's identification as the Messiah produced both Jewish opposition and Roman fear of political strife. Accordingly, Jesus was arrested, tried, executed by crucifixion, and buried by his followers.

The *New Testament* records that 3 days after Jesus's death, his tomb was found to be empty (*Mark* 16:1–7). Subsequently, Jesus is reported to have appeared to some of his followers who proclaimed that he had risen from the dead (*Matthew* 28:16–17). Christians vary in their interpretation of this event. Some accept Jesus's resurrection literally, whereas others understand it more symbolically or broadly as evidence of God's plan and power to establish a new era (*Acts* 2:23–24). Still other Christians emphasize that the resurrection event validated survival of the teachings of Jesus (*John* 16.8), or they stress that it is an expression of the hope that death can be overcome by God's power (*Romans* 6). Christians believe that their relationships with God were restored through Jesus as the Son of God who is regarded as both human and divine and a mediator between God and sinful human beings. The innocent suffering of Jesus and his death on the cross are considered redemptive by believers (*I Corinthians* 15:3).

Suffering in Christianity

Suffering, illness, and healing are important ideas in Christianity. Suffering, although not regarded as good in itself, may be redemptive; that is, it can deliver one from sin or its consequences as exemplified in Christ's crucifixion (Kitchel, 1986). In his ministry, moreover, Jesus healed the blind (*John* 9), those who were lepers (*Luke* 17:11-19), and others. The view of suffering for Christians, like those with other theistic beliefs, relates to an understanding of God and God's relationship with humanity. Several perspectives that explain why suffering exists can be found in the *New Testament* of the Christian *Bible.* One view, incorporated from Judaism, is that illness is a form of punishment (*I Corinthians* 11:27-32). Suffering results when God's will has been violated. Another view of suffering reveals the power of God to heal (*John* 9). Still another view of suffering is that it is a test of faith, a belief shared by some Jews as described in the *Old Testament Book of Job.* In the *New Testament,* Christians are reminded that suffering can be endured and transcended through faith:

> My dear friends do not be surprised at the painful test you are suffering, as though something unusual were happening to you. Rather be glad that you are sharing Christ's sufferings so that you may be full of joy when his glory is revealed (*I Peter* 4:12-13).

Thus, suffering may promote the spiritual growth of Christians and direct the sufferer's attention to that which is everlasting (*I Peter* 1:24-25).

Early Christians explained, but did not attempt to determine, a precise reason for suffering and evil. They regarded most suffering and evil occurrences as the consequence of the inappropriate use of personal freedom and free will resulting in sin; that is, separation from God (*Romans* 5). In some cases, however, illness was regarded as the result of personal sin (*John* 5:14) or demon possession (*Mark* 7:24-30). Stanley Hauerwas (1990) has observed that the modern desire to explain God's intention in allowing evil is influenced by the thinking of the Enlightenment, which emphasized rational explanations for phenomena. But in earlier times, Christians and others accepted the existence of evil in the world. This persistent Christian perspective eschews the need for a reasoned explanation of suffering and other evils. As summarized by Hauerwas, the Christian response has grown out of convictions rather than rational explanations. He writes:

> So Christians have not had a "solution" to the problem of evil. Rather, they have had a community of care that has made it possible to absorb the destructive terror of evil which constantly threatens to destroy all human relations (p. 222).

Consolation

Because many Christians do not rely on intellectual means for resolving the problem of suffering, sources of consolation must be discovered elsewhere. Their view is that suffering is real but transient. It is transformative because it has meaning in God's eternal plan. Even those persons who believe that suffering is the result of punishment seem more comforted than those who suffer for "no reason" (Hauerwas, p. 30). Many Christians find comfort in the teaching that suffering stimulates spiritual development. Paul's second letter to the Corinthians made clear that the spirit is able to survive suffering. His words are:

> For this reason, we never become discouraged. Even though our physical being is gradually decaying, yet our spiritual being is renewed day after day. And this small and temporary trouble we suffer will bring us a tremendous and eternal glory, much greater than the trouble (*II Corinthians* 4:16–17).

The Christian guide for enduring suffering is found in Jesus who was innocent yet suffered pain, crucifixion, and death with fortitude and without judgment (Sockman, 1961). In Jesus's suffering, Christians glimpse that which is universal and thus affirm that suffering can be overcome. They may experience God as a loving Father who cares for them and shares their suffering and whose love extends beyond death. These convictions comfort and imbue their suffering with meaning.

Health-care professionals who care for Christian patients should appreciate that their patients' faith establishes certain expectations for caregivers. First, there is a mandate to furnish care for those who suffer—the hungry, the thirsty, and the stranger without shelter—those who lack clothing, prisoners, and the sick (*Matthew* 25:35–39). Second, all persons are worthy of help, especially the poor or the least important (*Matthew* 25:40). Care for everyone is required because all are children of God, according to Christian belief, and, therefore, are worthy of help. Third, and finally, care needs to be compassionate and holistic. Although Jesus was a teacher and spiritual leader, he also charged his followers in the parable of the Good Samaritan to care for physical needs (*Luke* 10:29–35). Caregivers, therefore, are expected to be diligent, nonjudgmental, and sensitive to the Christian belief that God's Spirit is present in the "mortal body" (*Romans* 8:11). For most Christians, consolation comes from the sense that God's presence in Jesus Christ makes suffering endurable (Robinson & Johnson, 1982). Jesus's suffering on the cross makes it clear that suffering can be transcended and that the expectation of future joy makes suffering a "momentary affliction" (Raabe, 1989). St. Paul himself is an example of this Christocentric acceptance of suffering in the hope of joy to come after death (*Romans* 7:8).

ISLAM

Islam is a religion that was revealed to the Prophet Muhammad in Arabia in the 7th century. Followers of Islam are called *Muslims* (those who make their peace with Allah and man) (Ali, 1990, p. 4). They strive to submit to God's will and to do good to others. Muhammad was born in 570 CE (Eaton, 1985). His father died before he was born. As was the custom, his early years were spent apart from his widowed mother in the desert with his family, who were Bedouin nomads. Both parents and later his grandfather, who was his guardian after his mother's death, died before Muhammad was 8 years old. He was then nurtured by an extended family. In adulthood, he became a successful trader in Mecca (Esposito, 1991).

In his middle years, Muhammad began to seek solitude and time for reflection outside the city of Mecca, during which he had unusual spiritual experiences or revelations from God (Eaton, 1985). In an early revelation, the angel Gabriel is reported to have appeared to Muhammad and identified him as the true Prophet of God. At first reluctant, he became convinced of his mission, and he continued to have revelations from God throughout his life. Muhammad's teachings attracted followers, mostly among the poor initially, and also raised the suspicions of those in power. The opposition was related to Muhammad's attack on the established polytheistic religion and his claim to be a prophet of God (Esposito, 1991). He was persecuted, and when he learned of a plot to kill him and his followers, he fled to Medina where he eventually became accepted as a prophet. Muhammad conquered Mecca, united the Arabs and became a politically powerful person as well as the honored spiritual leader of many Arabs at the time of his death in 632 CE.

Basic Beliefs of Islam

The *Qur'an (Koran),* the scripture of Islam, is composed of Muhammad's revelations of the Word of God throughout his life as a spiritual leader (Rahman, 1966). The revelations that Muhammad conveyed came from God through the angel Gabriel. The *Qur'an* is regarded as the literal Word of God; it is not just a sacred book. Muhammad is venerated and understood to be the *agent* of Allah but not divine (Roberts 1981). The Word of God, according to the Muslims, had been revealed earlier to Adam, Abraham, Jesus, Buddha, and other prophets and also to some other righteous persons, but Muhammad's revelation is regarded as the final and authoritative one. Thus, previous revelations, religious leaders, and sacred books are acknowledged, but Islam is considered by believers to be the perfect revelation of God's Word (Roberts, 1981).

Islam is strictly monotheistic, and it also includes laws that regulate followers' behavior in considerable detail. Law is understood to be "the path in which God wishes men to walk" (Roberts, 1981, p. 54). Submission to Allah's will as defined by the *Qur'an* and other sources is required; sacred and secular laws are not differentiated as they are in the West (Sullivan, 1989). The distinguishing belief of Muslims is a briefly stated monotheistic creed, "There is no god but Allah and Muhammad is his Prophet" (Roberts, p. 36). This statement is the first of The Five Pillars of Islam that summarize the dedication of Muslims toward Allah. The others are (1) devotional worship and formal prayer (5 times a day), (2) obligatory tax for the needy, (3) fasting during the month of Ramadan, and (4) pilgrimage to the holy shrine of Mecca at some time in their lives (Roberts, 1981).

Consolation

Evil, illness, and suffering are among the problems that Islam addresses from the principles of the faith. Illness is generally understood to have natural causes. Allah is all powerful and may allow illness that has a divine purpose and is sent as a test of faith. God's mercy is also proclaimed and captured in the phrase, "In the name of God, the Merciful and Compassionate," that begins letters, lectures, and important matters (Esposito, p. 26). If the patient endures the suffering patiently, he may become a more faithful person (Rahman, 1987). In other cases, suffering is regarded as the consequence of sin; it is God's punishment. The proper response for the Muslim is to relinquish oneself to God (Sullivan, 1989). Muhammad is quoted as teaching surrender in illness:

> The Messenger of Allah—peace and blessings of Allah be on him—has said: "To say there is no might and no power except in Allah is a medicine for ninety-nine diseases, the least of them being anxiety." (Reported by Abu Hurairah, transmitted by Ahmad Friedlander, 1977, p. 138).

Although the preferred response to suffering is to trust Allah and patiently endure it, medicine is accepted by most Muslims. Allah is understood to heal through medicine according to the following quoted saying of the Prophet Muhammad:

> The Messenger of Allah—peace and blessings of Allah be on him—has said: "There is no disease for which Allah has not sent a cure." (Reported by Abu Hurairah, transmitted by Bukhari [Friedlander, 1977, p. 34]).

Muslim patients who are ill rely on faith and prayer but do not hope for a cure via a miracle like some Christians may seek. Although Allah is capable of performing supernatural miracles, Muslims believe that natural miracles and healing may occur through strong faith (Rahman, 1987).

Caring for a patient who is a Muslim requires that clinicians understand that all aspects of life—spiritual life and past and future actions—are inspired and guided by God and the Word of God revealed to Muhammad and recorded in the *Qur'an*. As Seyyed Nasr (1987) summarizes:

> It is the sound of the Qur'an which the newly born child first hears as the *Shahadah* is chanted into his or her ears . . .. And it is the Qur'an that is chanted at the moment of death and accompanies the soul in its posthumous journey to the Divine Presence (pp. 4–5).

It is to be expected, therefore, that the behavior and decisions of Muslim patients will be influenced by Islam's revelations and teachings. The significance of this foundation must be respected in all aspects of care.

Clinicians need to be aware that kindness is highly valued in Islam: "The Messenger of Allah—peace and blessings of Allah be on him—has said: 'He who is devoid of kindness is devoid of good'" (Reported by Jarir, transmitted by Muslim [Friedlander, p. 65]). Accordingly, the general mode of care should express this value. Additional guidance for clinicians may be found in the Islamic Code of Medical Ethics. It requires that patients be treated with dignity and not exploited, and that physicians recognize Allah's help in healing and acknowledge that medicine was created by Allah (Sullivan, 1989). Health-care professionals, moreover, need to be aware of the specifics of medical ethics that reflect the teaching and law of Islam in matters such as contraception, abortion, sexuality, genetic engineering, and death.

Care that reveals an understanding of Islam heals and prevents isolation and suffering. For example, offering the Muslim patient water for washing according to ritual before prayer is a sensitive act on the part of the caregiver (Roberts, p. 37). Dietary laws, especially the avoidance of pork, must be observed also. Patients who follow the Islamic spiritual life believe that suffering is part of the purpose of Allah. It must be accepted trustingly with the consolation that suffering is within the control of Allah who is all powerful.

SUMMARY

Suffering related to illness and disability may destroy patients' reasons for living. Suffering also may stimulate further examination of patients' life views and sustain or alter their perspectives on life. When ideology is destroyed, patients often appear to be passive and hopeless or victimized. As patients submit the suffering and its circumstances to review, they grapple with issues of its significance. For some patients, their religious orientation supports and sustains them in their struggles. It is incumbent on the clinician, therefore, to be respectful of the patients' religious beliefs, to provide support, and, more important, to avoid unintended harm. Sometimes it is helpful for both the clinician who furnishes direct care and the patient to enlist the competencies of other health-care professionals, such as chaplains and social workers, to furnish other perspectives on the patient's situation and to provide needed services.

Contact with that which is beyond the present or is everlasting diminishes loneliness, eases hopelessness, tempers vulnerability, and assuages loss in the midst of the chaos of illness and suffering. A caring manner communicates, "You are not alone" and "I will accompany you as you seek to make sense of what has happened." For health-care professionals, Buytendyk's (1990) perspective is useful. He writes, "The human body is always the corporeal being of a person with a soul" (p. 182).

The author wishes to thank Dr. Emmanuel Twesigye, Department of Religion, Ohio Wesleyan University, Delaware, Ohio, and Rev. Joseph Bracken, S.J., Xavier University, Cincinnati, Ohio, for their review of and suggestions for this chapter.

PRECEPT FOR PRACTICE

Suffering may evoke exploration of issues of existence, perspective, and meaning that can influence a patient's ability to accept, endure, and sometimes transform or overcome suffering.

REFERENCES

Ali, M. (1990). *The religion of Islam: A comprehensive discussion of the sources, principles and practice of Islam.* Lahore: The Ahmadiyya Anjuman Isha'at.

Bainton, R. (1966). *The horizon history of Christianity.* New York: Harper and Row.

Bareau, A. (1979). The experience of suffering and the human condition in Buddhism (J. Griffiths, trans.). In C. Geffre & M. Dhavamony (Eds.), *Buddhism and Christianity* (pp. 3–10). New York: Seabury Press.

Birnbaum, R. (1979). *The healing Buddha.* Boulder, CO: Shambhala.

Bowker, J. (1970). *Problems of suffering in religions of the world.* Cambridge: Cambridge University Press.

Buytendijk, F.J.J. (1957). The meaning of pain. *Philosophy Today, 4,* 180–85.

Chidwick, P. (1988). *Dying, yet we live: Our spiritual care of the dying.* Toronto: Anglican Book Center.

Cooper, B. (1989). Education for suffering and the shifting of the catena. *Religious Education, 84*(1), 26–36.

De Lange, N. (1986). *Judaism.* New York: Oxford University Press.

De Lange, N. (2000). *An introduction to Judaism.* Cambridge: Cambridge University Press.

Dossey, L. (1989). *Recovering the soul: A scientific and spiritual search.* New York: Bantam Books.

Doyle, D. (1992). Have we looked beyond the physical and psychological? *Journal of Pain & Symptom Management, 7*(5), 302–11.

Dumoulin, H. (Ed.). (1976). *Buddhism in the modern world.* New York: Collier Books.

Eaton, G. (1985). *Islam and the destiny of man.* Albany, NY: The State University of New York Press and the Islamic Texts Society.

Eisen, A. (1987). Covenant. In A. Cohen & P. Mendes-Flohr (Eds.), *Contemporary Jewish thought: Original essays on critical concepts, movements and beliefs* (pp. 107–11). New York: Scribner and Sons.

Encyclopedia Americana. (1996). Danbury, Conn.: Grolier.

Esposito, J. (1991). *Islam: A straight path.* New York: Oxford University Press.

Fox, D. (1987). Suffering and atonement as a psycho-Judaic construct. *Journal of psychology and Judaism 11*(2), 91–102.

Friedlander, S. (1977). *Submission: Sayings of the Prophet Muhammad.* New York: Harper and Row.

Good News Bible. (1992). New York: American Bible Society.

Gibbs, J.C. (1988). Three perspectives on tragedy and suffering—The relevance of near-death experience research. *Journal of Psychology and Theology 16*(1), 21–33.

Gilje, F. (1992). Being there: An analysis of the concept of presence. In D. Gaut (Ed.), *The presence of caring in nursing* (pp. 53–67). New York: NLN Press.

Glatzer, N. (Ed.). (1974). *Language of faith: A selection from the most expressive Jewish prayers.* New York: Schoken Books.

Hartman, D. (1978). Suffering. In A. Cohen, & P. Mendes-Flohr, (Eds.), *Jewish religious thought* (pp. 505–08). New York: Charles Scribner's Sons.

Hauerwas, S. (1990). God, medicine and problems of evil. In R. Neuhaus, *Guaranteeing the good life: Medicine and the return of eugenics* (pp. 216–28). Grand Rapids, Mich.: William Eerdmans.

Jurji, E. (1963). *The phenomenology of religion.* Philadelphia: The Westminster Press.

Kitagawa, J. (1989). Buddhist medical history. In L. Sullivan, (Ed.), *Healing and restoring: Health and medicine in the world's religious traditions* (pp. 9–32). New York: Macmillan.

Kitchel, J.C. (1986). The value of human suffering: Pope John Paul II and Karol Wojtyla. *Proceedings of the American Catholic Philosophical Association, 60,* 185–93.

Kushner, H. (1981). *When bad things happen to good people.* New York: Schoken Books.

Lamont, C. (1949). *Humanism as a philosophy.* New York: Philosophical Library.

Martin, M. (1990). *Atheism: A philosophical justification.* Philadelphia: Temple University Press.

Masutani, F. (1967). *A comparative study of Buddhism and Christianity.* Tokyo: Bukkyo Dendo Kyokai.

McDowell, J., & Stewart, D. (1989). *Spiritual Handbook of today's religions.* San Bernadino, Calif.: Campus Crusade for Christ.

Moore, T. (1992). *Care of the soul: A guide for cultivating depth and sacredness in everyday life.* New York: Harper-Collins.

Morrison, R. (1992). Diagnosing spiritual pain in patients. *Nursing Standard, 6*(25), 36–38.

Nasr, S. (1987). *Islamic spirituality.* New York: Crossroad.

Nouwen, H. (1972). *The wounded healer.* Garden City, NY: Doubleday.

Raabe, P. (1989). Human suffering in Biblical context. *Concordia Journal, 15*(4), 1–15.

Rahman, F. (1966). *Islam.* NY: Holt, Rinehart and Watson.

Rahman, F. (1987). *Health and medicine in the Islamic tradition: Change and identity.* New York: Crossroad.

Roberts, D.S. (1981). *Islam.* San Francisco: Harper and Row.

Robinson, H.W. (1939). *Suffering: Human and divine.* New York: Macmillan.

Robinson, G. (2000). *Essential Judaism: A complete guide to beliefs, customs, and rituals.* New York: Pocket Books.

Robinson, R., & Johnson, W. (1982). *The Buddhist religion: A historical introduction.* Belmont, Calif.: Wadsworth.

Schlesinger, G. (1989). The problem of suffering. In H. Schimmel, et al. (Eds.), *Encounter: Torah and modern life* (pp. 22–41). New York: Feldheim Publishers.

Singer, A. (1989). Human responses to suffering in rabbinic teaching. *Dialogue and Alliance, 3,* 49–56.

Sockman, R. (1961). *The meaning of suffering.* New York: Abington Press.

Speck, P. (1988). *Being there: Pastoral care in time of illness.* Great Britain, London: SPCK.

Spiro, M. (1970). *Buddhism and society: A great tradition and its Burmese vicissitudes.* New York: Harper and Row.

Starck, P., & McGovern, J. (Eds.) (1992). *The hidden dimension of illness: Human suffering.* New York: NLN Press.

Statistical Abstracts of the United States. (1998). Washington, DC: U.S. Department of Commerce.

Steeves, R., & Kahn, D. (1987). Experience of meaning in suffering. *Image: Journal of Nursing Scholarship, 19*(3), 114–16.

Sullivan, L. (1989). *Healing and restoring: Health and medicine in the world's religious traditions.* New York: Macmillan.

Varadhammo, V. (1996). *Suffering and no suffering.* Hindsdale, Ill.: Buddhadharma Meditation Center.

Watson, J. (1986–87). Suffering and the quest for meaning. *Loss, Grief and Care, 1*(1–2), 1975–88.

PART TWO

Care of the Sufferer

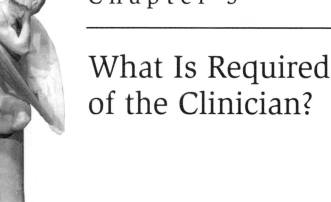

Chapter 5

What Is Required
of the Clinician?

No one can help anyone without becoming involved, without entering his whole being into the painful situation, without taking the risk of becoming hurt, wounded or even destroyed in the process.

HENRI NOUWEN (1972, P. 72)

The relief of suffering requires both professional and personal investment, as well as an exacting standard of clinical practice. Reprieves from suffering are most important when the illness cannot be cured. As death approaches, both the patient and the clinician become vulnerable in the clinical encounter.

Most patients expect their suffering to be recognized and relieved, or at least made more bearable. This expectation is a legacy of 18th-century thinking that held that rational and ethical persons who understand natural law would work to eliminate evils such as human suffering (Brinton, 1950). It is also a heritage of religious and philosophical views. More specifically, the 18th-century philosopher Emmanuel Kant (1969) contended that no less than moral law determines what *ought* to occur and that duty should direct practice. His guide for evaluating action was summarized briefly as: "Act so you treat humanity, whether in your own person or that of another, always as an end and never as a means only" (1969, p. 47). Applied to situations in which suffering exists, Kant's imperative directs health-care professionals to attend habitually to their duty of relieving suffering as well as supporting patients who suffer, never using that suffering for another purpose such as personal gain or organizational solvency.

To alleviate suffering or to help patients endure it, health-care professionals must first perceive and attempt to understand the suffering, respond competently and compassionately, and be willing to risk their own comfort level to provide care. "It is not possible," according to Dr. Janice Morse, et al., ". . . to avoid pain and still be compassionate. . ." (1992, p. 814). Where then does the motivation to experience emotional distress to relieve another's suffering come from?

Impetus to Relieve Suffering

> The test of a system of medicine should be its adequacy in the face of suffering . . .
>
> E. CASSELL (1991, P. VII)

The willingness or reluctance of health-care professionals to become involved in the suffering of a stranger is motivated by what they determine to be "right conduct." The way a clinician answers the question, "What is the essential nature of the patient?" reveals his or her standard of what is just and what constitutes appropriate care. On one hand, some will view the patient primarily as a physiological being who has experienced disease and disability. They will perceive that proper conduct, therefore, is to discover and competently apply ever more sophisticated scientific knowledge and techniques to manage pathology. On the other hand, for those clinicians who contend that a person responds to an illness as a thinking, feeling, social, and spiritual being, clinical and scientific competence alone do not suffice. Proper conduct for this group is to focus on understanding the patient's reality and needs and to formulate wise interpretations of that information.

According to Crane Brinton (1950), the former view is implemented with cumulative knowledge that has rapidly increased in quantity, and in which—particularly in the "hard" sciences—facts can be agreed on readily. In contrast, he maintains, noncumulative knowledge underlies the latter view. Knowledge of this type gathers more slowly, and ideas are subject to varied interpretations. The domain of noncumulative knowledge encompasses such questions that humans have posed for centuries without agreeing on answers: What is a person? What knowledge is real? and What is the right action? These are questions that have resisted absolute answers. Noncumulative knowledge is associated with a less definitive perspective of persons and right behavior.

Although these beliefs are extreme ends of the continuum, most clinicians do emphasize one conviction more than the other. At either end of the continuum, the perspective becomes too circumscribed to furnish a useful foundation for competent clinical practice. Purely scientific care may be insensitive whereas solely intuitive care may be uninformed, incorrect, or even dangerous. Although science-based care often furnishes cures, balance is required because the relief of the attendant suffering, which is often based on "soft" noncumulative knowledge, may be deprecated or even ignored as irrelevant.

The tendency of clinicians to avoid suffering by patients is a natural, even self-protective, inclination, but to be effective in suffering's relief, one must engage the patient because "Ultimately suffering is encountered one to one" (Byock, 1994, p. 9). To embrace the patient's suffering becomes the model to be sought, although the ideal is not always achieved. For Mother Theresa, the correct decision is both obvious and volitional. She writes, "It is only pride and selfishness and coldness that keeps us from having compassion" (Shield & Carlson, 1990, p. 151). Charity requires courage, however, to connect with the suffering of another because the suffering will affect the clinician's humanity. Attempting to comfort a dying patient anguishing over her abandonment by her family, for instance, may confront a clinician with the enormity of a hurt for which there is no balm.

What motivates and sustains those caregivers who involve themselves—beyond correct clinical care—in the suffering of others is their ability to establish a link with ideals and values that transcends the technologies and thus provides context and meaning for their professional practice. Even pausing to ask a preoperative trauma patient about his greatest concern reminds both patient and clinician of their shared humanity. Such caring moments transform the tasks of a job to a calling wherein a clinician may be invited into a life-defining crisis of a stranger and experience the fulfillment of enabling patients to endure the suffering or even surmount it. For Matthew Fox, this transformation of a job to a calling has a spiritual dimension that explains the clinician's fulfillment in spite of personal discomfort. He concludes, "When I am operating at my best, my work is my prayer. It comes out of the same place that prayer comes out of—the center, the heart . . .." (Shield & Carlson, p. 151).

Empathy: The Ability to Perceive Suffering

Agonies are one of my changes of garments
I do not ask the wounded person how he feels,
I myself become the wounded person,
My hurts turn livid upon me as
I lean on a cane and observe.
WALT WHITMAN (1940, P. 76)

The poet Walt Whitman, who was also a Civil War nurse, observed that humane caring recognizes the oneness of patients and caregivers. It requires the clinician to understand the patient's world, share the patient's feelings, and then initiate care. Warren Reich (1989) has defined empathy as ". . . the capacity to apprehend directly the state of mind of another person" (p. 106). In earlier times, the words *mercy, pity,* or *sympathy* may have been used in place of empathy; however, these terms are now often regarded as condescending or patronizing. Dr. Janice Morse, a nurse researcher and anthropologist, and her coauthors (1992) disagree. They argue that validating the patient's experience with such statements as, "This is a really difficult problem you have" or "I am sorry this happened to you," are appropriate intuitive responses that help a patient "get through" extreme suffering, often by opening dialogue (p. 812). She differentiated such responses, based on intuitive sensing of the patient's state, from responding with "therapeutic empathy," which can be learned and may be primarily cognitive.

Patients hope for empathy, along with compassion and competence, and consider it a large part of "good care." Moreover, empathy can have certain positive and practical outcomes for both the patient and clinician. When patients sense empathy, it invites them to share the narrative of their illness. It results also in better compliance with therapy, increased ability of the professional staff to tolerate difficult patient behavior, and opportunities to lower patients' expectations for unattainable outcomes (Zinn, 1993).

OBSTACLES TO ESTABLISHING EMPATHY

In spite of the apparent and inherent benefits, there are barriers to establishing empathy with patients. Sometimes health-care professionals assume authoritarian roles that shield them from recognizing their human commonality, the basis for empathy. In other cases, a "professional" style of detached interaction forms an obstacle to the establishment of empathy (Gould, 1990). Most significantly, and perhaps more commonly, the limited time available to interact with patients is a formidable barrier to developing empathy. An infrequently articulated consequence of recent changes in health-care financing is that the patient's time with health-care professionals has been rationed progressively. Hospital stays are now limited to that time required to treat acute physical problems or accomplish technical procedures. Organizational requirements often dictate that professionals treat more patients each day. In addition, minimally educated, unlicensed persons furnish more and more direct care. In many agencies, even caring and conscientious health-care professionals find their capacity for and opportunity to be empathic exhausted while patients experience the consequences of care without continuity and the effects of discharge before their human needs can be uncovered, often burdening their ill-prepared family to solve complex problems.

Certain patient characteristics, moreover, may make it difficult to establish an empathic relationship. Language barriers may preclude verbal communications. Persons from cultures that are significantly different from the culture of the clinician may generate little empathy and even misunderstandings. Stereotypes of groups such as the poor, elderly, and uneducated may interfere with the ability of health-care professionals to understand feelings of those who are different from themselves (Gould, 1990).

Another type of stereotype is diagnostic labeling that is employed commonly in health-care settings. Frequently, patients are referred to by their pathology, such as, "The bowel resection in 416." More ethically questionable is referring to a patient as "uncooperative" or "noncompliant" based on little or no data. Generally such terms really mean that the patient has a different agenda, based on dissimilar values, from that of the clinician and that these values are perceived to be more important by the patient than recommended therapy or treatment outcomes. Labeling often harms the patient, not only because it does not take into account the patient's relationships, experience, uniqueness (Mitchell, 1991), and right to self-determination, but also because other clinicians may accept the label, thus perpetuating the problem. Stereotypes and labels are comfortably simplistic and interfere with the motivation needed to discover a patient's unique perspective and manner of suffering and its causes.

Developing empathy requires a thoughtful health-care professional who is alert to a patient's suffering and its characteristics and the patient's need for empathy. The clinician may initiate the process even before meeting a patient by reading the clinical record to discover salient demographic factors, to determine how the patient has been impaired by the illness, and to review how the patient has responded. However, a cursory review of clinical information does not form the basis for empathy. The clinician must interact directly with the patient who becomes the receiver of the empathy (Barrett-Lennard, 1993, p 4).

CAUTIONS ABOUT ESTABLISHING EMPATHY

It may appear that empathy is always positive and a primary goal of care, but there are exceptions. Unduly focusing on empathy may be inappropriate when a patient has an urgent physical need. For example, it is more important to give priority to treating severe dyspnea than to assessing the patient's fear and distress. Empathy can sometimes interfere with the ability of a health-care professional to perform a procedure that inflicts pain, in spite of premedication.

It is important to recognize that empathy is morally neutral and that the clinician can use the knowledge gained from a patient for either good or for ill (Olsen, 1991). Manipulation of the patient by clinicians may result from misused information, leading to a course of action that may not be in accord with the patient's real wishes or best interests. This situation exemplifies Kant's prohibition against using persons as a means to an end. In summary, health-care professionals, although never able to fully comprehend a patient's suffering, may use empathy to briefly enter into the patient's isolation, hopelessness, vulnerability, and sense of loss. They have thereby honored and shared with the patient their mutual humanness.

Compassion: Sharing Suffering

> Compassion is thus the virtue by which we have a sympathetic consciousness of the distress or suffering of another person and on that basis are inclined to offer assistance in alleviating and/or living through that suffering.
>
> WARREN REICH (1989, P. 85)

For the health-care professional, empathy brings about cognitive awareness of suffering; however, that understanding needs to be communicated to and validated by the patient. Even when a health-care professional wishes to furnish compassionate care, the goal often proves elusive. Sarason (1985) attributed compassionless care for patients to deficiencies in medical education; however, the education of other health-care professionals may be equally lacking. He writes:

> . . . there is no focus in the medical curriculum on how students are aided to understand the nature, expression, and problematic aspects of the concepts of caring and compassion and to acquire the interactional skills of expression that begin to meet the criteria for caring and compassionate behavior (p. 61).

DIFFICULTIES OF COMPASSION

At a more basic level, acting compassionately may simply be a rather unnatural thing to do. Schlesinger (1989) observed that it is ". . . more remarkable for a man to act virtuously than selfishly" (p. 40). Because one must first empathize and encounter suffering to be compassionate, it does appear more common and self-protective to avoid it. Moreover, one cannot be guaranteed "success" by risking a meeting with a patient's suffering, for in some cases, suffering is inevitable and cannot be alleviated. Clinicians' only option may be to help the patient better endure the suffering (Lukas, 1986) or to prevent it when that is possible. Further, compassionate care often reveals itself to be a process rather than an event; thus, efforts may be regarded as unsuccessful and interactions abandoned prematurely by time-pressured health-care professionals or by early discharge practices.

Communication with patients may be both nonverbal and spoken. Health-care professionals who resist the temptation to flee from the suffering and are simply willing to spend a little time with the patient can communicate their sensitivity and caring. Without uttering a word, some clinicians are able to convey a sense of "presence" or "being there" in a way that the patient finds meaningful (Pettigrew, 1990, p. 503). According to Pettigrew, although little studied, presence appears to reduce the patient's feeling of isolation through a connection with the clinician that may continue even after he or she has departed. More typically, however, the establishment of a relationship depends on verbal interaction. It begins with attentiveness to what the patient has to say with the intention of comprehending, not just to gathering information about the world as the patient sees it (Barrett-Lennard, 1993). This phase has been described as *engagement* (Morse, 1992, p. 810) or *inducement* (Gallop, et al., 1990, p. 650). Communication that follows engagement focuses on understanding patients' perceptions of their worlds and communicating that understanding to the patient either verbally or nonverbally.

Well-intended health-care professionals are often immobilized when they initially encounter suffering, although they may wish to act compassionately. They may feel overwhelmed and pose such questions as, "How shall I act?" "What shall I say?" and "What shall I do?" (Drullinger, 1980, p. 60). In responding, it is helpful to be aware that there are two aspects of communication suffering persons use. The first has to do with the manner in which suffering is expressed, and the second aspect is the content (event or emotion) that is expressed.

Warren Reich (1989) has described three types of responses to suffering that are related to the manner in which patients express their suffering and clinicians respond. The first, "silent empathy, silent compassion," is often the best response to extreme suffering that cannot be articulated by the patient. Reich advised that it is important to be with the patient, withhold advice, be helpful, and be open to what the patient has to say. For example, one might say, "I can see that this diagnosis has been a shock. Is there someone whom I can call to be with you today?"Second, "expressive compassion," is a process that assists the patient to articulate his or her suffering and begin to understand and reformulate the experience. Finally, "having a compassionate voice of one's own" involves situations in which clinicians make themselves available as compassionate human beings to the patient while the patient resolves the distress and regains autonomy.

What is important is that the health-care professional learns what it means to suffer to determine what type of care is required. For example, a sick elderly person who has been abandoned by or who has outlived her family and friends (aloneness), who despairs of ever leaving the nursing home (hopelessness), who dreads increasing loss of independence (vulnerability), and who can find no meaning in her existence (loss) may be suffering more intensely and differently as a human being than her diagnoses of "status post fractured hip and congestive heart failure" would indicate.

FROM DATA TO PATIENTS' REALITIES

In general, interaction with such patients will include attention to the illness itself and to the patient's unique response to the illness. Experienced health-care professionals are often able to empathize quickly with the significant disability and the long-term rehabilitation that follows a cerebrovascular accident. However, sharing the patient's response to the illness episode and associated emotions is more difficult and less concrete for the health-care provider because feelings are integral to the individual's life view rather than to the nature of the pathology alone. Suffering may be identified when the characteristics depicted in the model of suffering exist (see Fig. 2–1).

While conversation about the pathology often requires the clinician to provide information or perform some activity, interaction that relates to the feelings or beliefs of the patient necessitates more personal involvement. Health-care professionals need to analyze patients' statements quickly and accurately during their interactions to be able to respond in a manner that supports patients and makes them feel understood. For example, there are several possible answers to a middle-aged patient who, following a stroke, says, "I won't be able to work again." The first type of response is, "Cheer up. You will feel differently when your condition improves." Although the clinician may correctly anticipate physical improvement, the patient has expressed the nature of his suffering (hopelessness, vulnerability, loss) and is not asking for information about his prognosis. Moreover, "cheer up" constitutes inappropriate reassurance that minimizes the patient's present distress. However well intended, this reply may be received as disinterest or rejection; no mutuality is established.

Another response by the health-care professional to the patient's statement might be, "You seem depressed about your future employability and independence." This reply correctly reflects the patient's emotional state and area of concern and establishes empathy based on an intellectual understanding of the patient's illness experience. Replies of this type have been described as therapeutic communication and can be learned (Morse, 1992). Yet another response by the health-care professional may be, "This must be a low point in your life. Much of who you feel you are seems to be related to your work." This response acknowledges the suffering and invites the patient to explore issues of meaning as well as practical concerns. It indicates that the clinician is attempting to share an understanding that goes beyond the articulated specific problem to the shared human need for self-definition and for meaning as well as for independence and financial security. Because the analysis is offered tentatively ("seems"), the patient is free to contradict it. If the analysis is correct, the patient may experience deep understanding. In a significant dimension of life, the patient feels understood, a feeling that may bring what one author has called "relief and connectedness" (Barrett-Lennard, 1993, pp. 5–6).

Articulated recognition of suffering establishes the intent to be involved in the suffering and also creates a bond between the clinician and the sufferer, according to Massignon (1989). Yet, no matter how empathic or compassionate the health-care professional may be, suffering, still to some degree, isolates patients and establishes a gulf between them and their caregivers. The sufferer can be further isolated by clinicians who are not aware of or humbled by the existence of this gulf and by the abiding enigma of suffering. Human suffering is infinite in the variety of its content and presentation. Its elusiveness cannot be underestimated because:

> . . . those who have known pain profoundly are the ones most wary of uttering clichés about suffering. Experience with the mystery takes one beyond the realm of ideas and produces finally a kind of muteness or at least a reticence to express in words the solace that can only be expressed by an attitude of union with the sufferer (Griffith, 1970, p. 26).

Caring

> Care begins when difference is recognized.
> A. FRANK (1991, P. 165)

While empathy enables health-care professionals to perceive patients' distress, sharing the feeling motivates them to initiate activity. The result of both is caring that is shaped by the identified characteristics of the individual suffering; the greater the patient's vulnerability, the greater the responsibility for caring. It is not a nicety added to technical skills. Caring is a perspective that grows out of an understanding of and respect for how a particular patient has experienced an illness. Caring is a moral imperative that is the core of professional practice. It begins with competence, may be observed in a variety of sensitive and attentive actions, and is best validated by the patient's human reaction.

CARING HAS BEEN DEVALUED

Although caring for the sick has ancient and honorable roots, the value of caring has been deprecated in modern health-care delivery. Centuries ago, Asklepios and his physician sons administered even to outcasts who suffered; thus, Homer regarded them as heroes rather than as mere craftsmen (Bailey, 1996). In caring for those who were otherwise rejected, however, these healers risked the wrath of the god Zeus by threatening his power to visit suffering on errant humans. Thus, unselfish and even self-sacrificial caring was established as a virtue of the ideal physician. In the West, the attribute of compassion was reinforced by Judeo-Christian teachings and by the philosophy of humanism, and it was incorporated as a value in organized medicine and in other health professions.

With the advent of scientific approaches to disease, however, many clinicians discovered that aligning with science-based curing functions furnished status, rewards, and power. Thus, claiming compassionate caregiving as a major component of clinical practice has become less valued. Today caring, as such, is not a reimbursable activity; therefore, it is often both invisible and unrewarded in the health-care system. Given the changes in health-care delivery, consistent caring is increasingly difficult to sustain, even in agencies with a philosophical or religious commitment to it. This virtue may be overwhelmed by the financial realities of the institutional budget and the pervasive philosophy and methods attendant to defining health care as a business. Institutional support for caring for suffering has too often been sacrificed to matters of efficiency and organizational profitability.

Inattention to the suffering of the person who is the patient has not vanquished suffering; rather, it has exacerbated the distress. Patients encounter the health-care system fearfully, typically regarding a symptom, a treatment, or a prognosis as a source of danger. Karl Jaspers, a psychiatrist and philosopher, has identified suffering as a limit or boundary situation that humans encounter in such specific situations as illness, struggle, and death (Ehrlich, 1975). Because these boundary situations ". . . elude the reflective and conceptual ordering of experience" (Schraq, 1971, p. 185), few patients are prepared to deal with such uncharted situations, and science offers no resolution. Consequently, such patients need to be enfolded in a mantle of caring because caring faithfully nurtures the patient's humanity, even when cure is not possible. It tells patients that they matter. What is required is caring as defined by Noddings (1984):

> To act as one-caring, then, is to act with special regard for the particular person in a concrete situation. We act not to achieve for ourselves a commendation, but to protect or enhance the welfare of the cared-for (p. 24).

CHARACTERISTICS OF CARING

This definition suggests several attributes of caring. First, health-care professionals should offer caring voluntarily and intentionally, identifying those patients who most need help and offering them competence and the gift of attention and time. Although caring is part of the defined clinical role, it goes beyond prescribed role-appropriate behavior and requires a willingness to enter into a quest to understand a patient's suffering, which is neither objective nor ultimately verifiable. Asking the patient, "What is this illness like for you?" affirms that the clinician is willing to be vulnerable to hear and share the patient's suffering (Schweizer, 1997, p. 16). Generally, patients will sense clinicians' receptiveness and express a problem that is of particular concern. Some patients will first test a clinician's sincerity by describing a "safe" problem, such as a physical discomfort. Other patients, particularly those without support systems, will immediately articulate a significant existential concern such as, "What will become of me?" In some cases, however, the clinician must draw on any available data and intuition because patients may find that articulating the suffering is difficult or impossible, or they may simply need to rest.

A second attribute of caring is paying attention to the patient's reality. It requires putting one's own values and perceptions on hold and attending to the patient's explanation of his or her own suffering and interpretation of what it means. It is necessary to grasp the essence of the suffering because it is the suffering in illness that may be healed or ameliorated as the pathology is treated, even if the therapy is unsuccessful. Perception of the patient's experience defines the unique needs and also the resources required to offer care. Suffering may first manifest itself as existential questioning, emotional distress, or a physical complaint. Application of scientific knowledge and techniques and skillfully tending to a patient's physical disorders communicates competence that engenders trust and a sense of security that invites patients to reveal their suffering. Even when suffering is mute, and cure is impossible, caring and comforting can be offered unfailingly to the sufferer.

Third, it is necessary to remember that care must benefit the patient. Sometimes caregiving can blur boundaries between the clinician and the patient, resulting either in undue influence of the clinician's values and goals or the clinician's control of the patient. When health-care professionals do not honor boundaries, the patient cannot remain unique. Caregiving can even be intrusive when silence is not honored. Caring can also go amiss when caring "recipes" are employed. Care of the sufferer should be particularized and regarded as a process extending over time, often involving a number of persons and approaches.

Fourth and finally, caring does not require cure. In fact, caring is most needed when cure is not possible.

Founded in the view that clinicians and patients are morally equal and undergirded by a willingness to be discomforted to help a stranger, caring does not require heroic gestures. In some chaotic and nonsupportive environments, health-care professionals must fight for just 10 minutes to devote to a sufferer. Yet, caring is marked mostly by ordinary small behaviors and attention to the manner in which services are rendered. Caring is a soft, comforting voice that invites the person who is the patient to connect with the person who is the clinician. Caring is eye contact. Caring is attentiveness often expressed by the clinician's leaning toward patients as they speak. Caring is anticipating patient's needs. Caring is performing intrusive procedures without causing unnecessary discomfort. Caring is shaving a patient's hairy arm before taping an IV. Caring is rewarming water during a bed bath. Caring is patting a patient's shoulder during anesthesia induction. Clinicians need not await the right time or hope for more time to be caring. Mostly, caring is a mosaic of behaviors that happens where we are. Such a view benefits patients and also clinicians who are frustrated by the constraints of the health-care system. "The self is saved or lost in how one acts toward others in small moments, not in what one decides about others in the big case conference" (Frank, 1992, p. 543).

THE COST OF CARING

> . . . without self-care the health care professional may lock his/herself in protective armor to shut out the pain, which risks shutting out the patient.
>
> R. PENSON (2000, P. 427)

To act with empathy, compassion, and caring exacts a toll on health-care professionals. In the extreme, the distress can lead to burnout, which is characterized by emotional exhaustion, treating people in an impersonal manner, and low accomplishment (Kash, et al., 2000). Burnout results from stress that has not been well managed over time, from a misfit between the clinician and the environment, and from discord between the clinician's expectations and reality (Weber & Jaekel-Reinhard, 2000).

It is necessary, therefore, that health-care professionals practice with a sense of self-awareness so that they can restore themselves before their distress negatively influences both their patient care and their personal lives. The daily stress of caring for patients who are suffering can often be relieved by respites such as coffee breaks during working hours, informal peer support, and pleasurable activities off duty. More prolonged and intense distress requires intentional activity that relieves stress. Some clinicians may find that art, music, or literature has a calming effect; others discover that physical activity or alternative therapies are helpful; whereas still other clinicians find meditation or prayer beneficial. In fact, one study of 261 nurses, house staff, and physicians working in a cancer center found that those who considered themselves religious had less emotional exhaustion and retained greater empathy for patients as compared with those who considered themselves not at all religious (Kash, et al., 2000).

Increased professional knowledge may modify clinicians' distress also. Sometimes developing better communication skills can make patient interactions easier and more helpful. More information about mental health issues or pain management, for example, identifies new approaches to care or signals the need for a referral to a specialist. This action not only benefits the patient, but also allows generalist clinicians to share the accomplishment of improving the patient's well-being. Knowing more about suffering—the goal of this book—will enable health-care professionals to perceive suffering as more manageable or amenable to relief.

When clinicians' distress is unrelieved and becomes progressive, burnout or even psychopathology may occur. In some cases, burnout may be related to clinicians' inabilities to find significance in their work (Pines, 2000). In other situations, the idealism that motivated clinicians' career choices is lost along with their sense of invulnerability (Alexander, 2001). Increasingly, managed care has become a significant cause of health professionals' distress. For example, a study of 2453 physicians found that arrangements that pressured them to practice in ways they did not consider appropriate engendered significant stress (Shapiro, 2000). Another study of 608 HMO physicians found that, "Perceived control over the practice environment was the single most important predictor of physician burnout" (Freeborn, 2001, p. 16). Thus, burnout can evolve not only from causes intrinsic to the work of caring for sick, suffering persons, but also from personal sources and extrinsic factors such as fiscally driven managed care.

Ongoing fatigue, diminished ability to concentrate, depression, addiction, and physical disorders such as insomnia and gastrointestinal problems are symptoms that signal the presence of burnout (Weber & Jaekel-Reinhard, 2000). Then clinicians usually need the support of mental health professionals to review their expectations, ways of coping, and sometimes future career paths because the distress is generalized. If they continue to practice, they often must withdraw from involving themselves in patients' suffering to focus their attention on resolving their own distress. In this case, the only expectation is that they will not cause suffering.

Other clinicians can relieve their daily stress and cumulative stress by self-awareness and intentional activity that furnishes energizing respites. They are capable of accepting Nouwen's challenge, "Who can take away suffering without entering into it?" (1972, p. 73). Health-care professionals who furnish direct care are in a unique position to identify and modify suffering because they have already established a relationship with the patient and, in many cases, these clinicians are able to prevent suffering.

When attending to suffering seems temporarily overwhelming, health-care professionals need to remember not to underestimate the simple. Small acts of human kindness that make the context of care less impersonal affirm the patient and relieve some suffering.

Clinicians also need to remind themselves that doing all that they can do to relieve suffering is enough. Limited time, energy, and other resources have always made it impossible to meet every suffering patient's needs, and these constraints will continue into the future. Realistic expectations enable health-care professionals to continue to encounter patients and to achieve potentially personal and professional renewal when they succeed in modifying suffering.

SUMMARY

Patients anticipate that health-care professionals will not only be competent, but will also be kind and enter into their distress and suffering while honoring their singularity. Clinicians are expected to be empathic, enabling them to perceive and to show understanding that the patient's human experience is inherent in illness. Relief may be possible when diligent caring begins with and is shaped by the nature of the patient's suffering. These expectations are met at a personal cost to health-care professionals who must be self-aware and intentional in managing their own distress. In the next chapter, selected causes of preventable suffering will be considered.

PRECEPT FOR PRACTICE

Health-care professionals who are willing to allow their humanity to touch patients' humanity are likely to attend to suffering in providing care.

REFERENCES

Alexander, D., & Klein, S. (2001). Caring for others can seriously damage your health. *Hospital Medicine, 62*(5), 264–67.

Bailey, J. (1996). Asklepios: Ancient hero of medical caring. *Annals of Internal Medicine, 124,* 2, 257–63.

Barrett-Lennard, G. (1993). The phases and focus of empathy. *British Journal of Medical Psychology, 66,* Part I, 3–14.

Brinton, C. (1950). *Ideas and men: The story of western thought.* New York: Prentice Hall.

Byock, I. (1994). When suffering persists. *Journal of Palliative Care, 10*(2), 8–13.

Cassell, E. (1991). *The nature of suffering and the goals of medicine.* New York: Oxford University Press.

Drullinger, D. (1980). *Compassion in the crisis.* Unpublished doctoral dissertation. Western Conservative Baptist Seminary.

Ehrlich, L. (1975). *Karl Jaspers: Philosophy as faith.* Amherst, Mass.: University of Massachusetts Press.

Frank, A. (1991). *At the will of the body: Reflections on illness.* Boston, MA: Houghton-Mifflin.

Frank, A. (1992). A medical ethic of suffering. *The Christian Century, 109*(May 20–27), 541–43.

Freeborn, D. (2001). Satisfaction, commitment, and psychological well-being among H.M.O. physicians. *Western Journal of Medicine, 174*, 13–18.

Gallop, R., et al. (1990). The empathic process and its mediators: A heuristic model. *Journal of Nervous and Mental Disease, 178*,(10), 649–54.

Gould, D. (1990). Empathy: A review of the literature with suggestions for an alternative research strategy. *Journal of Advanced Nursing, 15*,(10), 1167–74.

Griffith, J. (1970). The terrain of physical pain. In A. Paton, et al., *Creative suffering: The ripple of hope.* (pp. 25–37). Philadelphia: The Pilgrim Press and Kansas City, MO: The National Catholic Reporter.

Kant, E. (1969). *Foundations of the metaphysics of morals.* (L. Beck, trans.). New York: Macmillan.

Kash, K., et al. (2000). Stress and burnout in oncology. *Oncology, 14*(11), 1621–34.

Lukas, E. (1986). *Meaning in suffering: Comfort in crisis through logotherapy.* (J. Fabry, trans.). Berkeley, Calif.: Institute of Logotherapy Press.

Massignone, L. (1989). The transfer of suffering through compassion. In H. Mason (Ed.), *Testimonies and reflections.* (pp. 155–64). Notre Dame, Ind.: University of Notre Dame Press.

Mitchell, G. (1991). Nursing diagnosis: An ethical analysis. *Image: Journal of Nursing Scholarship, 23*,(2), 100–03.

Morse, J., et al. (1992). Beyond empathy: Expanding expressions of caring. *Journal of Advanced Nursing, 17*, 809–21.

Noddings, N. (1984). *Caring: A feminine approach to ethics and moral education.* Berkeley, Calif.: University of California Press.

Nouwen, H. (1972). *The wounded healer: Ministry in contemporary society.* Garden City, NY: Doubleday.

Olsen, D. (1991). Empathy as an ethical and philosophical basis for nursing. *Advances in Nursing Science, 14*,(1), 62–75.

Penson, R., et al. (2000). Burnout: Caring for the caregivers. *The Oncologist, 5*, 425–34.

Pettigrew J. (1990). Intensive nursing care: The ministry of presence. *Critical Care Nursing Clinics of North America, 2*(3), 503–10.

Pines, A. (2000). Treating career burnout: A psychodynamic existential perspective. *Journal of Clinical Psychology, 56*(5), 633–42.

Reich, W. (1989). Speaking of suffering: A moral account of compassion. *Soundings, 72*(1), 83–108.

Sarason, S. (1985). *Caring and compassion in clinical practice.* San Francisco: Jossey-Bass.

Schlessinger, G. (1989). Grappling with the problem of suffering. In H. Schimmel & A. Carmell (Eds.), *Essays on Torah and modern life* (pp. 22–41). Jerusalem: Feldheim Publishers.

Schraq, O. (1971). *Existence, existenz and transcendence: An introduction to the philosophy of Karl Jaspers.* Pittsburgh, PA: Duquesne University Press.

Schweizer, H. (1997). *Suffering and the remedy of art.* Albany: State University of New York Press.

Shapiro, R., et al. (2000). Managed care: Effects on the patient-physician relationship. *Cambridge Quarterly of Healthcare Ethics, 9*, 71–81.

Shield, B., & Carlson, R. (Eds.). (1990). *For the love of God: New writings by spiritual and psychological leaders.* San Rafael, CA: New World Library.

Simpson, J.A., & Weiner, E. (Preparers). (1989). *The Oxford English dictionary.* Oxford: Clarendon Press.

Weber, A., & Jaekel-Reinhard, M. (2000). Burnout syndrome: A disease of modern societies? *Occupational Medicine, 50*(7), 512–17.

Whitman, W. (1940). Song of myself. Part 33. In C. Morley (Ed.), *Walt Whitman: Leaves of Grass* (pp. 34–102) New York: Doubleday, Doran & Company.

Zinn, W. (1993). The empathic physician. *Archives of Internal Medicine, 153*(3), 306–12.

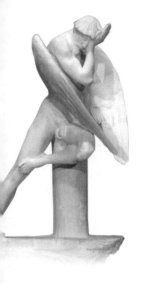

Chapter 6

How Can Suffering for the Wrong Reasons Be Prevented?

Suffering is given to the living, not to the dead . . . It is a man's duty to make it cease, not to increase it. One hour of suffering less is already a victory over fate.
ELIE WEISEL (1972, P. 315)

Suffering arises from two major sources: (1) disease or its treatment, or (2) thoughtless, incompetence, or unprincipled behavior encountered by patients. When patients present themselves for treatment and care, they may suffer because of a health-care professional's inconsiderate acts, inadequate pain relief, or circumstances that undermine their trust in the health-care system. Health-care professionals need to rectify situations within their purview—such as lack of courtesy—to prevent or minimize unnecessary suffering.

Discourteous Behavior

The greater the man, the greater courtesy.
J. PFORDRESHER (ED.) (1973, P. 903
[ALFRED LORD TENNYSON, *IDYLLS OF THE KING, THE LAST TOURNAMENT, LINE 228*])

Road rage, crude language, political attack ads, and an attitude of "anything goes" proclaim that a lack of civility exists commonly in contemporary society. Critics have devalued courtesy and good manners as inauthentic and a means of maintaining inequality among social classes (Karen, 1988). Current attitudes toward courtesy are often ambiguous, and for some persons "whatever works" is the operative rule for their interactions with others. Health-care environments are not immune from the attitudes and behaviors of the larger society.

EXAMPLES OF LACK OF COURTESY

Failing to recognize patients as fully human and violating their unique experience of illness is uncivil behavior that is inconsistent with the healing professions. For instance, failing to address patients by their appropriate name strips patients of their individuality. Showing disrespect is the 19-year-old patient-care assistant who calls the gray-haired bank president "Joe" or the assistant who calls a 90-year-old former music professor "Granny." Worse still, sometimes health-care professionals do not address patients at all, dismissing their humanity. "He has a lot of blood in his urine today," says a nurse, transforming a conscious and fully alert patient into a nameless object. Patients who are stigmatized by social class, culture, or homelessness, or those who have been injured or have injured others during a criminal act or while under the influence of drugs or alcohol, may suffer from lack of courtesy during their entire hospital experience. These examples validate Thomasma's (1995) observation that "Health care today is offered by strangers to strangers" (p. 20).

Care that is not civil disregards a patient's modesty and sense of privacy. Although it is likely that every nursing procedure book ever written includes the phrase, "Drape the patient for the procedure," this simple act of courtesy is frequently omitted in daily practice. In some situations, it is almost as if admonitions against unnecessarily exposing patients were a yet-to-be-discovered idea. As early as 1530, Erasmus wrote in *De Civilitate* on this subject:

> A well-bred person should always avoid exposing without necessity
> the parts to which nature has attached modesty. If necessity compels
> this, it should be done with decency and reserve, even if no witness
> is present. (Erasmus, 1530/1939, p. 103)

Care lacking in civility undermines patients' regard for the health-care institution, health-care professionals, and support staff and relegates patients to the status of objects. Appropriate professional attire is also a dimension of civility. When a middle-age engineer with severe chest pains enters an emergency department and encounters a caregiver wearing a tee shirt with a comic logo and another in jeans, dirty athletic shoes, and a rumpled lab coat, how will he judge the service to be rendered? The engineer fears for his life and must rely on

"Sue" and "Jim," the largest readable identification on the name badges, without really knowing the professional qualifications of either person.

Discourteous behavior not only breeches practice guidelines or etiquette rules—which may vary with time, place, and circumstances—but also, and more important, diminishes patients' trust, which is essential to their sense of safety and well-being. Feeling safe requires predictability, and when patients cannot fully control or anticipate the outcomes of a personal interaction (or of the illness), they feel insecure, vulnerable, or even fearful, and they suffer unnecessarily.

COURTESY AS MORAL CONDUCT

Buss (1999) has argued that courtesy is a moral issue. As she has elaborated:

> To treat someone "with respect" is to treat her in such a way that acknowledges her intrinsic value or "dignity." This is a value she has no matter what her deeds and accomplishments may be; it is tied to what she *is,* not what she *has done* (p. 796).

Courtesy, then, prescribes a view of human beings on which actions are based; it does not simply prohibit certain behaviors and advocate others. Therefore, courteous behavior is a means of expressing respect because it acknowledges the value of a patient, colleague, or other person; it is intrinsic to care and human interactions. Buss concludes that ". . . good manners are morally significant because they have symbolic significance . . ." (p. 807).

Addressing patients inappropriately or failing to include them in conversations is more than a misplaced attempt to be friendly or a lapse of attention; rather, such behaviors evolve from and symbolize a lack of respect for and deference to the patient's individuality and human vulnerability. Similarly, the failure to provide privacy shows lack of respect because it conveys that the sensitivities and boundaries of the other have been ignored (Carter, 1998). Likewise, the casual manner of dress of the two emergency department caregivers comes from the common view that clothing is a means of individual expression or is simply utilitarian. But sociologist Leoussi (1996) holds that denim conveys a casual attitude, unless it is required for strenuous work, and, "Rejection of aesthetically pleasing attire glorifies ugliness" (p. 101). Conventional, professional attire in patient-care situations fulfills the expectations of most patients (especially elderly patients). It bespeaks competence, and establishes that patient care is primary in the encounter—rather than making a statement of a clinician's individuality. Recognizing the effect of one's attire on patients sometimes requires restraint on the clinician's personal inclinations.

Courteous behavior is, in fact, moral conduct because it recognizes the mutual humanity of patients and clinicians. With colleagues, courtesy means recognizing the inherent worth of others. Keeping one's temper, disagreeing without being disagreeable, and offering criticisms based on factual information are all overt positive expressions of civility and courtesy. Sometimes courtesy even requires sacrifice of the clinician's immediate needs and desires to serve the greater good of patient confidence. Nevertheless, by modeling courteous behavior, health-care professionals can assume significant responsibility for establishing a clinical environment that recognizes the inherent dignity and value of every patient. Thus, the tired, schedule-driven professional who finds a moment to drape a patient for an intrusive procedure both subsumes her own needs to that of the patient and models civility. At a minimum, health-care professionals can view both courtesy and civility as acts of kindness because "Civility creates not merely a negative duty to do no harm, but an affirmative duty to do good" (Carter, 1998, p. 71).

Pain

> Every sentient being knows what it is to be in pain, but the true significance of pain eludes the most sapient. For philosophers, pain is a problem of metaphysics, an exercise for stoics, for mystics it is an ecstasy, for the religious a travail meekly to be borne, for clinicians a symptom to be understood and an ill to be relieved.
>
> C.F.W. ILLINGWORTH (1953, P. 9)

PAIN AS SENSATION

Inherent in the disease process is the phenomenon of pain. Pain's presence or fear of its occurrence is a common thread in patient distress that encompasses the themes of suffering. Effective management of pain or its total alleviation are primary goals in reducing suffering. For centuries, pain was regarded as mysterious, inevitable, and largely untreatable, although some efficacious substances such as the dried juice of the poppy (opium) were administered for pain relief from early times (Robinson, 1946). Historically, explanations of the etiology of pain with variations from culture to culture have been set forth. For the ancient Egyptians, demons were the source of pain; for the Indian Buddhists, pain was caused by the frustration of desire; and for the Chinese, pain was traditionally related to the balance of yin and yang (Bonica, 1991).

During the 19th century, the development of science led to the *organic* model of pain. According to Morris (1991) this model, ". . . tells us that pain, of every kind, is merely the result of nociceptive impulses traveling along neural pathways between the site of tissue damage and the brain" (pp. 282–83). This organic prototype evokes the optimistic view that the sensation of pain can be promptly and fully relieved and the corollary view that suffering is constituted by pain alone. Yet, the most casual perusal of the medical literature reveals that much pain is undertreated and goes unrelieved. For example, a study of 49,971 nursing-home residents found that 26 percent reported daily nonmalignant pain, whereas 25 percent of that group received no analgesics (Won, et al., 1999). Another study of nursing-home residents with cancer found that 37 percent had unrelieved pain and that 25 percent of the patients received no analgesics for daily pain (Bernabei, et al., 1998). These studies, and many others, validate that much pain is unrelieved, a fact that belies the implied optimism of the organic model and exposes the gap between theory and practice.

OBSTACLES TO PAIN RELIEF

Health-care professionals would furnish a higher standard of pain management if they recognized certain barriers to relieving pain. Perhaps the foremost obstacle to pain relief is the misconception that patients cannot report their pain reliably. Yet, *only* the patient experiences the pain and his or her reports must be accepted as valid. According to McCaffery (1972), "Pain is whatever the experiencing patient says it is, existing wherever he says it does" (p. 8). Nearly 3 decades later, Portenoy and Lesage (1999) again remind clinicians that "Because pain is inherently subjective, a patient's self-report is the gold standard for [pain] assessment" (p. 1695). However, clinicians may need to further assess some patients' expressions of pain. They may be influenced by ". . . culturally constructed notions about the meaning of pain that are embedded in the person's cognitive system . . ." and are often unconsciously held (Johnson, 1989, p. 28).

Sometimes patients themselves impose barriers to effective pain management. Those who experience pain may impede their own relief because they do not wish to appear weak by reporting their pain. Still others remain silent because they believe that pain is inevitably a sign of disease progression, which they do not wish to have confirmed. Sometimes families (and patients) minimize pain reports because they fear that addiction or confusion will follow medication. This situation may be especially true when family members are the primary caregivers. In other cases, health-care professionals may lack information about the most current treatment protocols or technology for pain management. They may fear causing addiction, or they may be overwhelmed by the complexities of pain management, particularly for patients with chronic pain or with multisymptom illnesses.

Regulation and the possibility of physician discipline by medical boards, insurers, or governmental agencies have been recognized as creating a culture that deters effective pain management. Although it has been estimated that only 5 percent of disciplinary actions pertain to overprescribed opioids (Martino, 1998), the perceived possibility of sanction and its financial and emotional consequences constitute a threat, even if the charges made are proved to be unfounded. When practice is questioned, investigative procedures that examine only dosage and length of use of an opioid—rather than the patient's condition and effectiveness of treatment—as indicators of the appropriateness of prescribing particular analgesics can cause great difficulty for both physicians and patients. Ideally, prescribing data needs to be interpreted by medical board members, attorneys, and consultants who are knowledgeable about pain management (Hyman, 1996).

IMPROVING PAIN RELIEF

The Pain Relief Act (PRA)—developed by the Project on Legal Constraints on Access to Effective Pain Relief of the American Society for Law, Medicine and Ethics—seeks to alleviate physicians' fears of inappropriate sanctions. Based on the duty to relieve pain, the PRA provides that health-care professionals cannot be prosecuted for providing pain-relief treatments that are within practice guidelines (Shapiro, 1996). In addition, some states have enacted legislation or pain statutes that limit legal sanctions when care is directed to pain relief. Furthermore, the U.S. Department of Health and Human Services Agency for Health Care Policy and Research released Acute Pain Management Guidelines in 1992 and Cancer Pain Management Guidelines in 1994 that define an acceptable standard of care for patients who experience pain. According to Shapiro, these guidelines, when applicable, may be employed in malpractice cases to validate an accepted standard of care.

A promising approach to better pain management is found in the standards of the Joint Commission on Accreditation of Health Care Organizations (JCAHO). These standards require that pain be systematically assessed and treated in health-care settings (JCAHO, 2000). The approach is expected to be multidisciplinary and requires prompt identification, evaluation, and treatment of pain. The standards also provide direction to increase professional knowledge about pain-relief interventions, educate patients in reporting pain and expecting its relief, evaluate and improve processes and outcomes, and develop policies to support the accomplishment of goals. Nevertheless, undertreating pain may continue to be silently rewarded for some time because this behavior is embedded in the health-care culture. Undertreating pain may still be considered unlikely to incur the risks or sanctions associated with perceived overprescribing. The status quo of undertreating pain may continue to be supported also by a broader cultural ethic that includes a fear of drug abuse, belief that pain should be endured stoically, and a general risk-avoidance stance of health-care personnel and institutions (Martino, 1998). This ethic needs to be transformed by intentional changes in the curricula for health-care professionals and in the culture of health-care institutions.

CONSEQUENCES OF INADEQUATE PAIN RELIEF

Inadequate pain relief is obviously not benign. Reporting on a decade of research at the City of Hope National Medical Center, Ferrell (1995) indicated that poor pain control resulted in increased patient symptoms such as fatigue, anorexia, sleeplessness, constipation, and nausea. Lang (1999) concluded that "Pain can induce numerous metabolic and neuroendocrine responses. While seemingly homeostatic, these changes can have significant physiologic and sometimes adverse consequences" (p. 14). Chapman (1984), writing even earlier about postoperative pain that is unrelieved, noted that upper intra-abdominal or thoracic pain results in muscular splinting, impairment of ventilation, and ultimately pneumonitis—and increased morbidity or even death for patients in poor physical condition. In contrast, he noted, ". . . a narcotic-induced analgesia results in improvement of ventilation" (p. 1268).

Pain as a Human Experience

> Disease can destroy the body, but pain can destroy the soul.
> EDWIN LISSON (1987, P. 649)

The organic model of pain, as discussed in the foregoing section, is clearly dominant in health-care practice. It regards pain as a sensation and suggests that total relief is possible, if not fully realized. By comparison, little in medical literature addresses pain as a human experience and a dimension of suffering beyond the sensation. Yet pain is interpreted and typically articulated by the patient as "my pain," signaling that pain is experienced uniquely. Thus pain and its management becomes a complex issue for the health-care professional. Pain of unknown origin, prolonged or chronic pain, pain of terminal illness, and undertreated pain—in particular—are related to patients' perceptions, past experiences, and manners of coping with life's critical events. There is, moreover, not only personal uniqueness but also cultural variability in relation to beliefs about pain and how it should be perceived, expressed, or relieved. When the experience of pain evokes the beliefs of the model of suffering presented in Part I of this work (I am alone, I feel hopeless, I am vulnerable, or I have experienced a loss) in a context of fear or anxiety, pain ceases to be only an organic phenomenon; it becomes suffering.

FEAR

> Pain has but one acquaintance and that is death.
> EMILY DICKINSON (POEM NO.1049,
> JOHNSON [ED.,1865/1960, P. 479])

As Dickinson observed, pain often evokes the fear of death and, for many patients, its attendant terrors. Conversely, when pain is relentless and unendurable, patients may welcome death as a means to end the pain. Even if the pathology that is the source of the pain will not end existence, it causes patients to realize that they are finite creatures and that their lives will be altered and constrained temporarily or permanently. They may no longer possess a sense of assurance that their cherished goals can be achieved, and, consequently, fear that the future of their lives is without a predictable course.

Some fears associated with pain have been identified by researchers. Strang (1997) studied 78 cancer patients and found that ". . . the overall mean pain score and the mean worst pain correlated significantly with concerns and fear about the future, worries about the pain, and fear of pain progression and anxiety" (p. 303). Ferrell's (1995) research that focused on the meaning of pain for the patient diagnosed with cancer included fear. She found that "Pain meant the patient had cancer and if the pain increased, the derived meaning was that the cancer had recurred or was progressing" (p. 17). Another study of patients with chronic back pain (Crombez, et al., 1999) investigated the pain-related fears among 104 patients. Findings revealed that the fear was more disabling than the pain; that is, ". . . pain-related fear is a precursor of disability, rather than the consequence of it" (p. 338). Supportive care seeks to remove the fear in accord with Montaigne's (1580/1958) advice, "I shall be in plenty of time when I feel the pain, without prolonging it by the fear of pain. He who fears he will suffer already suffers what he fears" (p. 840).

The patient in pain not only has a hurtful sensation but also must live with and through the pain experience hour by hour. Pain evokes fears of disease progression and of more pain and even of death, which may have negative physiological and emotional consequences. People experience pain and the associated fear differently. A cancer patient (Frank, 1991) summarized it this way, "Fears vary. Differences in fears are part of the individual experience of illness, and care is about recognizing differences" (p. 43).

ISOLATION

> When he could bear no more, the pain kept on.
> The sore made him squeal and scream for somebody to come.
> Nobody ever came.
>
> PHILOCTETES [HEANEY (1990, P. 38)]

In this play by Sophocles (c. 496–406 BCE), the Greek chorus related Philoctetes' feelings of utter abandonment and mute suffering when he was deliberately marooned on the island of Lemnos with a painful, ulcerated, and rotted foot that was the consequence of a snake bite (Heaney, 1990). Philoctetes' feelings of separation and despair could be expressed today by some patients who also suffer because their cries for pain relief go unheard when their family and friends have abandoned them in their suffering or when clinicians do not even ask about pain or evaluate its relief. When clinicians are unable to judge patients' pain accurately and then delay or undermedicate, provide few comfort measures, or take no action at all, patients suffer. In part, this situation occurs because the nature of pain is difficult for patients to express adequately.

According to Scarry (1985), "Physical pain does not simply resist language, but actively destroys it, bringing about an immediate reversion to a state anterior to language, to the sounds and cries a human being makes before language is learned" (p. 4). Thus,

Philoctetes squealed and screamed as a wordless (or mute) expression of his pain and agonizing aloneness. It is the responsibility of clinicians to help patients find ways to express their pain, if only through visual analog scales or pain questionnaires that furnish descriptors, and thereby assuage their isolation. Patients who cannot express themselves or who are not heard by clinicians experience further isolation and alienation that result in increased pain and suffering. Describing his experience with cancer, Frank (1991) wrote, "Pain that is inexpressible isolates us, to be mute is to be cast out by others" (p. 34).

HOPELESSNESS

> Pain—has an Element of Blank
> It cannot recollect
> When it began—or if there were
> A time when it was not.
> EMILY DICKINSON
> (JOHNSON [1865/1960, P. 760])

When pain seems endless, hope fades and suffering is intensified. Often the patient who has not had adequate pain relief believes that relief cannot be achieved. Quality of life may deteriorate, and patients may request euthanasia or consider suicide. Chronic, unrelenting pain that is either related to progressive disease or that lacks a demonstrable underlying pathology is particularly difficult for patients and clinicians. The pain itself becomes the essential problem. As cure becomes elusive, patients begin to perceive that the pain will last indefinitely. This perception is reported in the *Old Testament* of the *Bible* through the account of Job's travails, as cited previously. Assailed with a plague of boils, hopelessness overtook him, and he lamented, "The night racks my bones and the pain that racks me knows no rest" (*Job* 30:16–17).

Clinicians must be alert to the possibility that patients who experience hopelessness will develop a major depressive disorder (MDD). Bottomley (1998) quotes Hughes as saying that this condition is one ". . . in which mood and vitality is lowered to the point of despair. Patients report that life is meaningless, and experience feelings of misery and hopelessness" (p. 181). Health-care professionals who are generalists need to know several things to identify such situations. First, MDDs commonly coexist with physical disorders. For example, Lander et al. (2000) have estimated that 20 to 50 percent of terminally ill cancer patients have depressive disorders (p. 337); van de Weg et al. (1999) contend that approximately 500,000 of 2 million stroke survivors experience post-stroke depression (p. 269).

Second, although comorbid depression is often unrecognized, it has significant consequences for patient well-being. For example, in stroke patients, untreated depression seems to be associated with increased disability, according to van de Weg et al. For cancer patients, untreated depression may result in reduced compliance with therapy, longer hospitalizations, decreased quality of life, and greater mortality (Newport & Nemeroff, 1998).

A valid diagnosis of MDD requires a specialist, but other clinicians need to be aware that there is a greater likelihood of MDD when certain conditions exist. Bottomley (1998) has identified that corticosteroid administration, chemotherapy, whole brain radiation, endocrine disorders, and paraneoplastic syndromes are potential organic sources of depression. Patients who have family problems and lack social support are at greater risk for depression (Lander et al., 2000) as are those who have had a history of psychiatric disorders or certain personal characteristics such as a high need for control (Pirl & Roth, 1999). The authors assert that "The most common cause of depressed mood in cancer patients is uncontrolled pain" (p. 1296).

Third, generalist clinicians must be aware that they are the ones most likely to identify a possible MDD and to initiate a referral to a mental-health professional for further evaluation. Treatment may include psychosocial approaches such as psychotherapy or pharmacotherapy (Newport & Nemeroff, 1998), or in some cases, a combination of approaches. Identification and treatment of depression are often successful in improving patients' quality of life and in enhancing their physical well-being. When the precise manner in which a stressor initiates depression is better identified, more effective treatment is anticipated, according to Newport and Nemeroff (1998).

The consequence of not recognizing depression is significant because hopelessness may become desperation, an agonizing form of suffering. The loss of hope may even result in a desire for relief through death. Fishbain's (1999) review of 18 studies from 1966 that correlated pain with suicide ideation, attempts, or completion, in fact, concluded that unrelieved pain must be regarded as a suicide risk factor. Thus, providing pain relief and having mental-health professionals available when needed is part of the imperative to relieve suffering. Without such care, "Hope can be utterly smothered by the heavy, suffocating, and totally mind-dominating desire for death when pain and distress are relentlessly intense and unending" (Roy, 1998, p. 3).

VULNERABILITY

> . . . the worst thing in the body is pain.
> ST. AUGUSTINE, *SOLILOQUIES*
> (OATES, C. 387 bce/1948, P. 271).

As noted previously, patients with pain are at the mercy of health-care professionals for pain alleviation. When clinicians do not evaluate the patients' pain sensations and experiences accurately, pain relief and comfort measures are doomed to be inadequate. "Being in pain," wrote a sufferer, "is to be constantly reminded that you are alive and trapped in your body" (Lum, 1997, p. 65). Patients, therefore, may grow to distrust the competence of caregivers, feel abandoned, and experience a loss of self-sufficiency as the unrelieved pain increases their vulnerability and limits what is possible for them to accomplish or to endure. Clinicians have a moral obligation to prevent pain when possible or to treat pain within the limitations of available knowledge and resources, thereby relieving both hurt and suffering. Empathically perceiving the pain is not enough because perception alone does not necessarily make clinicians compassionate or competent to judge pain intensity or to furnish effective pain relief (Watt-Watson et al., 2000). Thus, it is critical to individualize the suffering and to *do* something skillfully until the pain is modified or relieved. The persistence of unrelieved pain, failure to prevent it, and unnecessary suffering it causes constitute an unacceptable standard of practice for health-care professionals.

LOSS

> When the body breaks down, so does life.
> A. FRANK (1991, P. 8)

Pain causes sufferers to recognize that life and all that is significant to them may be extinguished by the injury or disease that they are enduring. Whether objectively true or not, ". . . pain is a metaphor for death for both patients and family members" (Ferrell, 1995, p. 612). Pain challenges patients to identify or discover a way of making sense of their suffering because the organic model of pain has no inherent meaning; however, unrelieved pain is exhausting and impedes the search for meaning. Patients' beliefs about pain and suffering are largely framed by their personal experiences, religious or philosophical views, and cultural mores. Although most patients attach some meaning to their pain and suffering, some are unaware of that meaning; therefore, they experience their situations as meaningless. Given the abyss that looms, some patients despair whereas others struggle to affirm or find significance that may furnish perspective and also comfort. As a young priest dying of cancer wrote, ". . . so often in our lives, the very situation that causes so much pain or sorrow is the very place that we can experience God's blessing and new life" (Willig, 2001, p. 4).

Although health-care professionals have been encouraged consistently to relieve pain, there is an exception when an occasional patient, who has made a considered judgment to endure pain, is encountered. For example, in Christian tradition certain ascetics used "sacred pain" to link them to the divine (Glucklich, 1999). In this tradition, a few patients choose to endure their pain and suffering as Christ did and to offer it up to God (or to a higher power) for others' redemption. Willingly bearing pain, according to this tradition, provides meaning for such patients. Clinicians should be mindful of not interfering when the process is recognized because the belief links the patient with that which is eternal and unchanging and beyond the pain. However, in some cases, pain relief may be respectfully offered as a brief respite that some patients will accept, particularly at night. Otherwise, pain relief for patients who wish to make a sacrifice or restitution or to grow spiritually through necessary suffering should not violate their autonomy.

SUMMARY

Patients who experience unrelenting pain both hurt and suffer unnecessarily. Health-care professionals must possess the will and competence to relieve the sensation of pain. In reviewing clinical research on pain, one finds that the studies in which patients experienced limited or no pain relief far outnumber those that document good pain management.

Although suffering may not always be associated with pain, commonly it is ensnared in pain or in the anticipation of it; thus, good pain-management skills are necessary. In most cases, managing pain begins by controlling the sensation, guided by the following three maxims:

1. Believe the patient's account of pain.
2. Relieve pain promptly and persist until the patient confirms that it has been relieved. Substandard treatment of pain is negligent care. Avoid rationing analgesics and unwarranted concern about addiction. Be alert to the need to monitor pain level and adjust medication.

3. Recognize that administering analgesics does not necessarily match control of pain for the patient. Additional treatment modalities may be required or the health-care professional needs to attend to the patient's pain as a human experience (Wall & Melzack, 1994).

Minimizing the transformation of pain to suffering is critical, especially when pain persists. First, help patients regain their sense of control and diminish their vulnerability by demonstrating that the pain can be reduced or eliminated and that other symptoms can be relieved. Patients who feel better usually suffer less. Second, relieve ambiguity and anxiety or fear by identifying the source of the pain, as well as describe the treatment plan and side effects. Third, recognize that pain exists in a context of concerns, emotions, individual history, attitudes, and culture that influence pain behavior and meanings. Fourth, provide opportunities to discover how patients interpret their pain and recognize that explanations may change over time.

Sometimes, patients' outlooks may not be congruent with the views of their family, clinicians, or others (Ferrell, 1995). Regard pain as a symbol that may represent the humanity of the patient for "Not relieving pain brushes close to the act of willfully inflicting it" (Morris, 1991, p. 191).

PRECEPT FOR PRACTICE

Health-care professionals have it within their power to minimize or prevent suffering by treating patients as moral equals and by relieving or managing pain expertly.

REFERENCES

Bernabei, R., et al. (1998). Management of pain in elderly patients with cancer. *Journal of the American Medical Association, 279*(23), 1877–82.

Boncia, J. (1991). History of pain concepts and pain therapy. *Mt. Sinai Journal of Pain Therapy, 58*(3), 191–202.

Bottomley, A. (1998). Depression in cancer patients: A literature review. *European Journal of Cancer Care, 7,* 181–91.

Buss, S. (1999). Appearing respectful: The moral significance of manners. *Ethics, 109,* 795–826.

Carter, S. (1998). *Civility: Manners, morals and the etiquette of democracy.* New York: Basic Books.

Chapman, C.R. (1984). New directions in the understanding and management of pain. *Social Science and Medicine, 19*(12), 1261–71.

Crombez, G., et al. (1999). Pain-related fear is more disabling than pain itself: Evidence on the role of pain-related fear in chronic back disability. *Pain, 80,* 329–39.

Erasmus (1530). De Civilitate. In Norbert, E. (E. Jephcott, trans.) (1939/trans. 1978) *The civilizing process: The history of manners.* New York: Urizen Books.

Ferrell, B. (1995). Impact of pain on quality of life: A decade of research. *Nursing Clinics of North America, 30*(4), 609–24.

Ferrell, B., & Dean, G. (1995). The meaning of cancer pain. *Seminars in Oncology Nursing, 11*(1), 17–22.

Fishbain, D. (1999). The association of chronic pain and suicide. *Seminars in Clinical Neuropsychiatry, 4*(3), 221–27.

Frank, A. (1991). *At the will of the body: Reflections on illness.* Boston: Houghton-Mifflin.

Glucklich, A. (1999). Self and sacrifice: A phenomenological psychology of sacred pain. *Harvard Theological Review, 92*(4), 479–506.

Good News Bible. (1992). New York: American Bible Society.

Heaney, S. (1990). *The cure at Troy: A version of Sophocles Philoctetes.* London: Faber and Faber.

Hyman, C. (1996). Pain management and disciplinary action. *Journal of Law, Medicine and Ethics, 24,* 338–43.

Illingworth, C.F.W. (1953). *Peptic ulcer.* Edinburgh: E & S Livingstone, Ltd.

Johnson, T. (1863/1865/1960) (Ed.). *Emily Dickinson: Complete poems.* Boston: Little, Brown and Company.

Johnson, T. (1989). Contradictions in the cultural construction of pain in America. In C. Hill & W. Fields (Eds.), *Drug treatment of cancer pain in a drug oriented society* (pp. 27–37). New York: Raven Press.

Joint Commission on Accreditation of Health Care Organizations. (2000). *Pain assessment and management: An organizational approach.* JCACO Publishers.

Karen, R. (1988). Revenge of the wounded. *The Yale Review, 78,* 85–96.

Lander, M., et al. (2000). Depression and the dying older patient. *Clinics in Geriatric Medicine, 16*(2), 335–56.

Lang, J. (1999). Pain: A prelude. *Pain Management, 15*(1), 1–16.

Leoussi, A. (1996). Keeping up appearances. Clothes as a public matter. In D. Anderson (Ed.), *Gentility recalled: Mere manners and the making of social order* (pp. 97–106). London: The Social Affairs Unit and the Acton Institute for the Study of Religion and Liberty.

Lisson, E. (1987). Ethical issues related to pain control. *Nursing Clinics of North America, 22,*(33), 649–660.

Lum, G. (1997). Prisoner of pain. In Young-Mason, J., *The patient's voice: Experiences of illness* (pp 63–73). Philadelphia: F.A. Davis.

Martino, A. (1998). In search of a new ethic for treating patients with chronic pain: What do medical boards do? *Journal of Law, Medicine and Ethics, 26,* 332–49.

McCaffery, M. (1972). *Nursing management of the patient with pain.* Philadelphia: JB Lippincott.

Montaigne, M. (1580/1958). *The complete essays of Montaigne.* (D. Frame, trans.). Stanford, Calif.: Stanford University Press.

Morris, D. (1991). *Culture of pain.* Berkeley, Calif.: University of California Press.

Newport, D., & Nemeroff, C. (1998). Assessment and treatment of depression in the cancer patient. *Journal of Psychosomatic Research, 45*(3), 215–37.

Oates, W. (Ed.). (1948). *Basic writings of Saint Augustine,* Volume I. New York: Random House.

Pfordresher, J. (Ed.). (1973). *A variorum edition of Tennyson's Idylls of the King.* New York: Columbia University Press.

Pirl, W., & Roth, A. (1999). Diagnosis and treatment of depression in cancer patients. *Oncology, 13*(9), 1293–1306.

Portenoy, R., & Lesage, P. (1999). Management of cancer pain. *Lancet, 353,* 1695–1700.

Robinson, V. (1946). *Victory over pain: A history of anesthesia.* New York: Schuman.

Roy, D. (1998). The relief of pain and suffering: Ethical principles and imperatives. *Journal of Palliative Care, 14*(2), 3–5.

Scarry, E. (1985). *The body in pain: The making and unmaking of the world.* New York: Oxford University Press.

Shapiro, R. (1996). Health care providers' liability exposure for inappropriate pain management. *Journal of Law, Medicine and Ethics, 24,* 360–64.

Strang, P. (1997). Existential consequences of unrelieved cancer pain. *Palliative Medicine, 11,* 299–305.

Thomasma, D. (1995). Beyond autonomy to the person coping with illness. *Cambridge Quarterly of Health Care Ethics, 4,* 12–22.

Van de Weg, F., et al. (1999). Post stroke depression and functional outcome: A cohort study investigating the influence of depression on functional recovery from stroke. *Clinical Rehabilitation, 13,* 268–72.

Wall, P., & Melzack, R. (1994). *Textbook of Pain.* Edinburgh: Churchill Livingstone.

Watt-Watson, J., et al. (2000). The impact of nurses' empathic responses on patients' pain management in acute care. *Nursing Research, 49*(4), 191–200.

Weisel, E. (1972). The accident. In S. Rodway (trans.), *The night trilogy.* (pp. 205–318). New York: Hill and Wang.

Willig, J. (2001). *Lessons from the school of suffering.* Cincinnati, OH: St. Anthony Messenger Press.

Won, A., et al. (1999). Correlates and management of nonmalignant pain in the nursing home. *Journal of the American Geriatrics Society, 47,* 936–42.

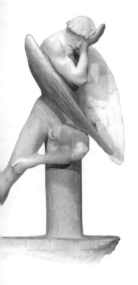

Chapter 7

How Is Erosion of Trust a Source of Suffering?

Trust and integrity are precious resources, easily
squandered, hard to regain.

S. BOK (1978, p. 249)

It is unrealistic to advocate that attention to human suffering in illness
is critical without recognizing the factors in managed care that limit
the ability of health professionals to furnish compassionate care.
According to Brother Ignatius Perkins,

> . . .the threats on clinicians in being restricted in their practices and
> moved to the role of technicians threatens the integrity of the
> patient-professional relationship in new and disturbing ways. . . .
> The end or telos (of health care) is healing of the person, even when
> the patient should succumb to the disease, not the improvement of
> the financial profiles of third-party payors (Personal communication,
> June 7, 2001).

The most significant consequence of this shift in emphasis from
healing to financial solvency is the erosion of trust that some patients
experience and others suspect. In this chapter, specific causes of
skepticism, or distrust, as a source of vulnerability unrelated to the
disease and the effect it has on patient suffering are discussed.

When patients suffer from a critical illness, their confidence in the
health-care system is tested most severely; however, it appears that
even perspective patients have diminished faith and confidence in the
present system. Their feelings may range from being "on guard" to
feeling outright antipathy and suspicion. In part, this change is
because of patients' greater educational attainments, readily available
information sources, and negative media reports. In addition, some
patients and future patients have become skeptical as a result of their

own or others' illness experiences and have concluded that too much trust will place them at risk.

Along with incivility and poorly managed pain, erosion of trust in the current health-care system is potentially a preventable cause of suffering. Some people identify managed health care, defined as ". . . a system of health-care delivery that tries to manage the cost of health care, the quality of that health care, and access to that care" (Kongstvedt, 1996, p. 996), as the primary source of suspicion. In 1999, for example, about 400,000 Medicare patients lost access to the health-care provider to whom they had entrusted their well-being when some HMOs withdrew from the market because of increased costs and limited federal reimbursement (Benjamin, 1999). Still other patients have become doubtful about new managed-care arrangements, restrictions on physician and treatment choice, and the motives of for-profit health-care plans. Scholars, moreover, have questioned the justification for managed care (Pelligrino, 1986), analyzed the risks of dismantling the professional ethic of beneficence (Angell, 1993), and identified that a business model for health-care service inappropriately dominates in the health-care system today (Macklin, 1993).

It is beyond the scope of this work to discuss the strengths and weaknesses, the varieties of managed-care organizations (MCOs), and the many current issues in health-care financing and delivery. Evaluation is both conceptually and methodologically difficult, but it seems clear that patients' trust and confidence in the system have deteriorated. Health-care professionals have many concerns of their own, and they recognize patients' doubts about whether the system can be relied on in their time of need. This perception is important because lack of trust creates feelings of susceptibility to harm, in addition to those vulnerabilities inherent in the illness experience itself. Although most payment plans for health care are managed to some degree, a cost-driven model, rather than a care-driven model, can result in more suffering.

Issues of Trust

"Trust can be defined here as the extent to which organizations and clinical personnel are perceived to be functioning in the best interests of patients and the public, acting as their agents and advocates for their needs and welfare" (Mechanic & Rosenthal, 1999, p. 284). Trust presumes that one party, the truster, is dependent on another, the trusted, for help with something of value (Baier, 1986). Patients are inherently vulnerable because their wholeness has already been damaged by illness, they lack the expertise to heal themselves, and they may be unable to advocate for themselves to negotiate a complex system. Without such jeopardy, trust would be unnecessary. Ill persons need assistance and commit their care and therapy to clinicians, health-care plans, and institutions that have great discretion and power. Patients' faith is well placed if that power is employed to their benefit rather than misused for ends such as increasing organizational profitability. In some cases, "Persons with diminished autonomy stand in need of protection" (Macklin, 1989, p. 27). Methods may even be employed to hide the misuse of power, thus permitting abuse to continue (Baier, 1986). Such action violates the patient's expectation of goodness, regarded as ". . . a demand—a tacit demand—not to betray the expectations of those who trust us" (Lagerspetz, 1998, p. 5). The traditional relationship of trust is fiduciary; that is, it is one in which patients can experience assurance and confidence.

Trust includes confidence in persons based on a belief, developed through an extended relationship, in the integrity of another person who furnishes direct care. Trust includes, also, confidence in systems, usually based on lengthy experience (Seligman, 2000). In the current system, however, many patients must switch their physicians and be hospitalized according to the dictates of health insurance plans, sometimes contrary to patients' wishes. "Trust begins where prediction ends," according to Lewis and Weingert (1985, p. 976). Abuse of trust results in anger, the authors note, when an emotional bond with a person has been broken, and litigation may occur when patients' trust in a system has been abused. Further, such mistreatment may result in increased external scrutiny and greater regulation of a system. The long-term consequences of abuse of trust are severe because ". . . trust in some degree of veracity functions as a *foundation* among human beings; when this trust shatters or wears away, institutions collapse" (Bok, 1978, p. 31).

UNCERTAINTY ABOUT COMPETENCE

Competence in furnishing care and treatment is a patient's minimal expectation; yet many are uneasy about the quality of care available. Their concerns have been fueled by media reports of high-profile malpractice cases as well as by a general increase in reporting errors perpetrated in hospitals and other practice settings. A growing number of patients perceive that their care has been substandard, or they have personally experienced errors. Until recently, reports of adverse events often related to a clinician's lack of knowledge. For example, a study over a 7-year period of patients with appendicitis misdiagnosed by inexperienced physicians found that such patients ruptured their appendixes 91 percent of the time, resulting in more extensive surgical procedures and postoperative complications (Rusnak, et al., 1994) as well as in more suffering.

Recent interest in system-related factors that contribute to errors has been incorporated into research studies with increased frequency. For instance, one investigation of sources of errors that were self-reported by physicians found that clinical factors, such as premature focus on one diagnosis or treatment as a source of error, were equal in significance to physician stressors, such as feeling hurried (Ely, et al., 1995). Similarly, a recent study of errors in chemotherapy administration found that 63 percent of the 186 well-educated nurse respondents described 140 errors within 1 year. Most errors (39 percent) related to wrong dosage, 22 percent of the patients involved required medical intervention, 10 percent needed prolonged hospitalization, and 1 death was reported. Workplace factors that contributed most to the errors were identified as stress and understaffing (Schulmeister, 1999). Without increased resources, it can be expected that over time such contextual conditions will continue to be a major source of errors and patient harm. As such errors receive greater publicity, patients may become more fearful and anxious and thus more prone to personal suffering.

Rationing Practices

As the distinction blurs between managing the delivery of care and managing care, patients point to the health-care delivery system itself as the source of diminished quality of care. For example, decreased reimbursement levels and increased regulatory requirements contribute to the burnout of health-care professionals because of understaffing, particularly in hospitals where patient acuity seems to be ever increasing and length of hospital stays diminishes. This phenomenon of brevity of contact with professionals and restricted care undermines the very system designed to provide healing. Further, MCOs have been regarded as providing less-than-desirable care because of the existence of planned limitation of patient access to potentially beneficial services. MCOs' use of specific strategies that restrict care has been identified precisely by some enrollees but are mostly unknown to patients. According to Field and Cassel (1997) these strategies include:

- Limiting benefits furnished
- Using financial incentives to providers to furnish less care
- Requiring approval of certain services in advance
- Limiting care available via the use of practice guidelines
- Employing productivity requirements to limit time with patients
- Increasing the cost of using out-of-plan providers
- Making specialist referrals difficult to obtain

Some of these aforementioned strategies are not unique to MCOs, and not all MCOs use each of them; however, taken as a whole, these strategies do ration care. For example, limiting access to specialists—particularly those who are out of the MCO network—reduces costs, but the care provided by a generalist may be less effective than that provided by a specialist (Mechanic, 1996). Care furnished by a physician extender that requires a physician's knowledge and skill, or care by a generalist physician that needs the expertise of a specialist results in what Pelligrino (1997) has termed ". . . the creep of incompetence" (p. 327). This incompetence can result in delayed or missed diagnoses, complications, and other problems. Whether the claim that MCOs can improve care outcomes—particularly those that are significant but intangible—at reduced costs is uncertain and not easily subject to validation. In the meantime, enrollees become skeptical about quality when care is denied or unnecessarily delayed, when they discover that they have not, by policy, been informed about potentially beneficial treatment options, and when their autonomy is overshadowed by imposed standardized care and by bureaucratic procedures. Thus, patients lose their trust in the system and its clinicians and feel increasingly vulnerable, which increases suffering.

In some cases, withholding certain services is the consequence of the intrusion of administrators or other nonmedically educated third parties into significant medical recommendations (Gray, 1997). In general, the law holds that unlicensed persons may not direct medical care (Hall, 1988). Although some directives from unlicensed persons are advisory and allow physicians to make final decisions, clear financial incentives in MCOs often influence the physician's choice among alternatives. Binding directives pertaining to care policies, sometimes formulated by unlicensed persons, mislead patients about who actually made the decision that a physician communicates. Physician managers may reduce the foregoing problem if they have freedom to decide a course of action based on medical science and patient requirements. The generic problem when systems explicitly ration care, according to Hall, is that "Federal policy makers are operating under the misconception that we can save money without

sacrificing either the quality or quantity of medical services delivered"
(p. 499).

Broader issues of promoting care quality, given the foregoing
situations, have received attention also. Ruskin (1997) has supported
the concept of vicarious liability for MCOs under the doctrine of
respondent superior defined as "let the master answer" (Thomas,
1997). He has argued that MCOs substantially direct physicians'
practices through control of expenditures using devices such as
binding practice directives and established capitation rates.

Havinghurst (2000) has asserted that health-care plans have not
met the goal of improving quality of care and reducing costs. In his
view, there is a lack of management methods to improve the quality
of care. For example, selected subcontractors, who are the actual
suppliers of services, make rationing decisions that affect patients
based primarily on financial incentives. He concurred that the
concept of vicarious liability is relevant because MCOs actually
supply care through physicians and other health professionals and
agencies. This view would make health plans, with certain
exceptions, responsible for patient injuries because plans can exercise
power that influences care decisions. Havinghurst has argued also
that because health-care plans have considerable power to manage
care, they have an equal responsibility to furnish care of high quality,
justifying the concept of vicarious liability. Public discourse on issues
of competent care and attendant problems is warranted even though
it will increase a patient's sense of vulnerability. Such discussion is
urgently needed.

Waning Loyalty to Individuals

Perhaps patients' distrust of competence is best captured by Bloche's
(1999) identification of a paradigm shift in patients' consent from ". . .
prophylaxis against clinical actions contrary to patients' interests to
justification of professional authority to weigh the interests of others
over those of the patient" (p. 271). In a reverse "Robin Hood" method
of health-care delivery, MCOs place some subscribers at risk to benefit
others and maintain plan solvency. According to Churchill (1997, p.
120), "This happens by design, not by accident. . . ." The inherent
ethical dilemma adds to the burden of professionals who are also
highly distressed and more error prone because of constraints of
understaffing and imposed standards of productivity. Some patients
may sense the clinician's shift in loyalty, which may precipitate
distrust. This shift can be related to overzealous rationing of costly
treatments, deception about how some treatment decisions are made,

and failure to disclose treatment alternatives not provided by a health-care plan.

In general, health-care plans do not equally reward cost containment and the provision of personalized, high-quality care. Indeed, Dudley, et al. (1998) argued that plan income should be related to the quality of care provided. The problem of implementing this principle is that, although some indicators of quality exist, quality of care is a complex phenomenon that resists precise evaluation. The authors, therefore, validated the distrust of some patients concerning care for profit when they concluded that ". . . when quality is hard to measure, there are many ways to increase return on equity by lowering quality" (p. 655).

DOUBTS CONCERNING HONESTY

The inequality of power between vulnerable human beings who are patients and health-care professionals, financing plans, or institutions should impose certain moral obligations on the provider, among which is honesty. Patients normally wish to make health-care decisions ". . . *in terms of our own personal values, beliefs and experiences* [author's emphasis]" (Wear, 1993, p. 35). Such choices require that health professionals provide information that is complete and truthful and that they reveal the real character of health-care plans and systems. Unfortunately, it seems that not only increasing numbers of patients doubt the credibility of both health agencies and payors, but some patients express complete distrust of them, particularly patients whose health status requires increasing dependence on the existing system.

Withholding Information

Two sources of lack of faith related to concealing salient medical information serve as examples. First, it is reported that some MCOs impose "gag rules" on their physician employees. Sometimes, these rules prevent physicians from speaking negatively of the plan or require them to withhold information about the value of treatment not provided by the plan. Additionally, the plan may require that designated expensive treatment options may not be discussed with patients until they are preapproved for that patient (Brody & Miller, 1998). When advice about a better treatment option or a more effective medication not in the MCO's formulary is withheld, patients are even denied the possibility of using their own resources to purchase a more effective product or treatment outside the plan. In some cases, the option to enroll in a less limited health-care plan is also unavailable to the patient. Veach (1991) regards physicians' role as gatekeepers to be a serious problem because it recasts the patient-physician relationship as though the Hippocratic oath had been rewritten thus:

> Warning all ye who enter here. I will generally serve your interests, but in the case of marginally beneficial expensive care, I will abandon you in order to serve society as its cost-containment agent (p. 20).

A second situation that generates patient distrust is failure of some MCOs to reveal physician financial incentives. Most patients are aware that in traditional fee-for-service plans, physician income may be enhanced by providing more services—some of which have been criticized as unnecessary. It appears that fewer persons are aware that financial incentives also relate to limiting services in MCOs. A portion of the physician's income in an MCO may be put at risk if capitated expenditures exceed the anticipated limit. In other situations, a bonus may be offered if the plan operates at less than the expected cost (Kongstvedt, 1996). Thus, the physician's self-interest may be justified, resulting in the curtailment of the use of expensive resources such as certain diagnostic studies or treatments, hospitalization, or specialist consultation. Such highly cost-conscious care achieves worthy political and social goals or increases the profitability of the plan—depending on one's perspective.

Deterioration of the Fiduciary Ethic

Cost-containment arrangements may compromise the ethic that has historically undergirded the physician-patient relationship. Traditionally, patients have relied on the principle of benevolence, wherein they could confidently expect physician loyalty to their best interests. According to Angell (1993), some physicians not only are now agents for their patients, but also serve society's interest in determining whether the value of a particular patient's treatment is worth the cost to society; that is, they are double agents. The author has written that this dichotomy undermines physicians' central mission, which is fidelity to healing the individual, a mission that is central to other health professions as well. When patients discover that physicians are not free to act in their best interests, trust in their physicians is extinguished—and, by extension, their reliance on the integrity of the health plan or institution is surely compromised or even destroyed altogether.

As indicated previously, sometimes strategies to limit care to achieve financial and social goals are not revealed to patients or are briefly explained by general statements published by the plan. When patients experience the attendant problems, feelings of anger and betrayal emerge because "The worst lie of omission belongs to the category of lying, which is concealing by pretending to reveal" (Brown, 1998, p. 113).

Bloche (1999) has argued that the assertion that both individual patient-care goals and social goals can be met simultaneously by physicians is in error and is consequential for patients. Such an erroneous view, according to Bloche,

> . . . neglects, even denies the affective experience of the victim of (physician) infidelity—the person who trusts and is betrayed and is thus intimately wounded by another person. Quite apart from any adverse health consequences, the physician's infidelity violates another, often when the other is most vulnerable (p. 272).

Angell (1993) has summarized the perception that the health-care system cannot be entrusted to benefit patients by writing, "In short, can it be that the ethical underpinnings of the practice of medicine have been scrapped in a single decade for financial reasons? Is economics driving ethics?" (p. 280).

DIMINISHED RESPECT FOR INDIVIDUALS

Trust is engendered when patients believe that their unarticulated demands for respect and their expectations of goodness are recognized (Langerspez, 1998). Care that is impersonal is the antithesis of respectful care. Patients are aware that spending adequate time with clinicians to be seen as persons in need of healing has diminished. The change from earlier practice is due to understaffing, to delegation of care to minimally educated persons, to record keeping demands that assure reimbursement, or to productivity quotas that intentionally ration patients' contact with health-care professionals. Diminished patient contact makes establishing and sustaining an ongoing human and therapeutic relationship difficult for patients and health-care professionals alike. For example, in hospitals, well-educated nurses have witnessed the transformation of their professional competencies into a collection of tasks delegated downward to unlicensed personnel with a few weeks of training for whose actions they are responsible.

In general, more and more care is delivered by persons with less and less training. Physicians and other professionals, who by virtue of prolonged education, commitment, and temperament, wish to incorporate patients' inner experiences of illness into their care are impeded. Their professional time is diverted to tasks such as seeking approval from a health-plan functionary to hospitalize a patient, determining which drugs are included in a particular formulary, and attempting to establish which regulation applies currently. As a result, many clinicians suffer role deprivation, change jobs or career paths, or plan to retire at the earliest possible date. This situation may increasingly deprive patients of the wisdom and skills of the most experienced health-care professionals.

In some cases, depersonalization has been institutionalized as the norm. For example, critical pathways or care maps may be used to plan care for hospitalized patients. The pathways or maps include a series of condition-specific tasks and progress indicators and have been touted as promoting both efficiency and quality. According to Vezeau (1997), the larger purpose of this planning and intervention strategy is to assure that patients use only the anticipated resources and are discharged within the time allocated by the Diagnosis-related Group (DRG). Used prescriptively rather than as guides, such standardized tools require neither patient input nor that a relationship with the patient be established to validate or to modify and individualize the plan. Often, it is difficult to incorporate consistently into standardized plans even such relevant additional factors as the coexistence of other illnesses or frailty due to age.

Additionally, lack of regard for the privacy of patients' medical records makes patients aware that respect for them has been violated or is at risk. Although many patients presume that their right to privacy is virtually sacrosanct, their illusions may end abruptly. For example, when a newly diagnosed patient with diabetes begins to receive unsolicited advertising by companies that sell diabetic supplies, she knows that her diagnosis has been shared with commercial interests. She may also have good reason to feel vulnerable concerning future insurability or possibly negative employment ramifications. Although health-care providers must protect patient confidentiality, violations of confidentiality by insurers are not ordinarily illegal (Bloche, 1997). Use of patient information obtained to pay claims for commercial purposes is both common and unethical and has been regarded as a ". . . health privacy crisis" (p. 16) by the National Committee on Vital and Health Statistics (Etzioni, 2000). Several urgent reforms have been recommended including patient identifiers that make information, other than that required for direct care, unrecognizable to other parties. Yet, satisfactory patient privacy legislation has been difficult to formulate, approve, and implement.

Managed Death

Perhaps the ultimate loss of respect for the meaning and significance of the life of another rests in the notion of managed death, particularly the death of those considered to be an economic burden. Although the use of life-sustaining therapies has been a decision traditionally made by patients or their surrogates, some clinicians now report instances wherein they have been pressured to withhold treatment. In other situations, information has been presented to patients or families in such a way as to promote agreement that such therapies be withheld. Sprung, et al. (1997) have specified the concern that financial incentives sometimes play a role in foregoing life sustaining therapies, contrary to the real wishes of patients or surrogates. A more bleak possibility, set forth by Sulmasy (1995), is that if voluntary euthanasia or assisted suicide were legalized, some families would be manipulated to agree to active euthanasia for vulnerable patients. He concludes that, "Euthanasia for such patients would be in the best financial interests of all levels of management—the government, the HMO and the physician" (p. 135). Further, Sulmasy predicts, "The conflict of interest created by trying to make the physician both the agent of care and the agent of cost containment will come to a climax once HMOs begin to provide euthanasia and assisted suicide" (p. 134).

Contractual Thinking

In a general sense, trust in clinicians and institutions has been undermined because relationships built on trust have been replaced by contractual relationships. Patients could once feel respected by clinicians and institutions with whom they had experience and thus trusted; now, however, a contractual way of thinking has arisen in an atmosphere of mistrust and become the norm in an often impersonal health-care system (Baier, 1986). The contractual approach initially took the form of general consent to treat provided on hospital admission and informed consent for specific procedures. Consents of this type were based on potential issues of battery related to required touching and negligence in adhering to professional standards (Hall, 1993). Although some instruments may omit information concerning treatment alternatives or the option of nontreatment, informed consent of this type tends to preserve respect for patient autonomy.

A more thorny contractual issue, particularly for patients enrolled in MCOs, is prior "economic informed consent" (Hall, 1993, p. 656). Because patients delegate spending decisions to insurers and physicians, they lose much autonomy; therefore, it is argued that some type of consent is required. Types of implicit consent to limit payment for certain services have been identified by Hall (1993). They include:

1. Presumed consent—the patient would have agreed if he had been asked.
2. Bundled prior consent—a decision to enroll in the plan constitutes delegating treatment decisions to the medical director or treating physician.
3. Waiver of informed consent—enrollment in a plan inherently waives the right to be informed of rationing mechanisms.
4. Arbitration of specific disputes (Hall, 1993).

The author recommends against such silent rationing and advocates, "Some global disclosure to patients of rationing incentives, rules, and mechanisms is required at the onset of enrollment . . ." (p. 663).

Although some contractual relationships serve specific purposes, Hall's thoughtful analysis of some of the issues of managed care (1988, 1993) has raised questions about a contractual mode of thinking. Baier (1986) argues that such thinking is inherently flawed because contracts typically assume a relationship among or between persons of equal power. Little trust is required because expectations are explicit and violations can be identified easily. Illingworth (2000) adds that the context of contract development may include mutually agreed-on efforts to embellish quality, instances of bluffing and strategies to put a positive spin on some situations. These strategies, although relatively common in business, are inappropriate when the availability and quality of health care is being negotiated by parties whose power is unequal.

Contracts between patients and insurers or providers include one party, the patient, who has limited power. Therefore, patients have greater vulnerability because they are less knowledgeable and able to evaluate care, they are putting their health—something precious—at risk, and they may be impaired by illness when they are required to enter into a contract. Baier, an ethicist (1986), argues that contracts have become "the moral norm" (1986, p. 348) in health care, superceding trust. She has proposed a moral test for trust that, in her opinion, many contractual relationships with patients would fail. She advocates that each party in the relationship should be aware of what the other relies on to sustain the relationship. In her words:

> A trust relationship is morally bad to the extent that either party
> relies on the qualities of the other which would be weakened by the

knowledge that the other relies on them . . .. I have assumed that most people in most trust situations will not be content to have others rely on their fear, their ignorance and their spinelessness (pp. 255–56).

Fully substituting a legalistic, contractual paradigm for fiduciary relationships, therefore, undermines respect for the vulnerable person who is the patient and may result in what Pelligrino (1991) has termed "ethical minimalism" (p. 79).

In conclusion, patients are immensely vulnerable and dependent on health-care providers and payors to use their greater power to act to benefit them. Patients' trust can be abused by substandard care, by giving priority to some goal other than healing the individual, and by dehumanized care. Although patient rights legislation may resolve some of the most egregious abuses, it is not designed to restore trust. Thus, "Medicine without trust becomes marred by suspicion, fear and even danger" (Jackson, 1996, p. 196), and suffering is born.

SUMMARY

The potential to cause suffering by increasing vulnerability exists inherently in the current health-care system. The trust of patients— particularly those who are highly dependent on health-care personnel, agencies, and payors—has been eroded because of uncertainties about provider competence, questions about honesty, and diminished respect for individuals. These situations, to a greater or lesser degree, constitute the milieu in which care is delivered and become part of the patient's reality and illness experience. Patients can suffer because they are denied potentially beneficial care or because their humanity is negated by bureaucratic, productivity-driven systems. With an understanding of the situations that lead to an erosion of trust and greater patient vulnerability, health-care professionals may better modify the consequences of suffering that are system generated and exist in addition to the suffering intrinsic to the disease. As informed citizens, clinicians can be a knowledgeable voice advocating change.

PRECEPT FOR PRACTICE

Health-care financing and delivery systems that evoke concerns about competence, honesty, and respect for individuals can damage a patient's sense of trust and thereby contribute to increased vulnerability and suffering.

REFERENCES

Angell, M. (1993). The doctor as double agent. *Kennedy Institute of Ethics Journal, 3*(3), 279–86.

Baier, A. (1986). Trust and antitrust. *Ethics, 96*(2), 231–60.

Benjamin, G.R. (1999). Medicare HMO exodus: System correction or prediction? *Physician Executive, 25*(1), 77–78.

Bloche, M. (1999). Clinical loyalties and the social purposes of medicine. *Journal of the American Medical Association, 281*(3), 268–74.

Bok, S. (1978). *Lying: Moral Choice in Public and Private Life.* New York: Pantheon Books.

Brody, H., & Miller, F. (1998). The internal morality of medicine: Explication and application to managed care. *Journal of Medicine and Philosophy, 23*(4), 381–410.

Brown, A. (1998). *Subjects of deceit: A phenomenology of lying.* Albany, NY: State University of New York Press.

Churchill, L. (1997). Damaged humanity: The call for a patient-centered medical ethic in the managed care area. *Theoretical Medicine, 18,* 113–26.

Dudley, R., et al. (1998). The impact of financial incentives on quality health care. *Milbank Quarterly, 76*(4), 644–86.

Ely, J., et al. (1995). Perceived causes of family physician's errors. *The Journal of Family Practice, 40*(4), 339–44.

Etzioni, A. (2000). Medical records: Enhancing privacing, preserving the common good. *The Hastings Center Report, 29*(2), 14–23.

Field, M., & Cassel, C. (Eds.). (1997). *Approaching death: Improving care at the end of life.* Washington, D.C.: National Academy Press.

Gray, B.H. (1997). Trust and trustworthy care in the managed care era. *Health Affairs, 16*(1), 34–49.

Hall, M. (1988). Institutional control of physician behavior: Legal barriers to health cost containment. *University of Pennsylvania Law Review, 137*(431), 431–536.

Hall, M. (1993). Informed consent to rationing decisions. *Milbank Quarterly, 71*(4), 645–68.

Havinghurst, C. (2000). Vicarious liability: Relocating responsibility for the quality of medical care. *American Journal of Law and Medicine, 26,* 7–29.

Illingworth, P. (2000). Bluffing, puffing and spinning in managed care organizations. *Journal of Medicine and Philosophy, 25,*(1) 62–76.

Jackson, R. (1996). *A philosophical exploration of trust.* Unpublished doctoral dissertation. Lansing, Mich.: Michigan State University.

Kongstvedt, P. (1996). *The managed health care handbook.* Gaithersburg, Md.: Aspen Publishers.

Lagerspetz, O. (1998). *Trust: The tacit demand.* Boston: Kluwer Academic Publishers.

Lewis, D., & Weingert, A. (1985). Trust as a social reality. *Social Forces, 63*(4), 967–82.

Macklin, R. (1989). Ethical principles, individual rights and medical practices. *International Forum, 25*(Fall), 25–27.

Macklin, R. (1993). *Enemies of patients.* New York: Oxford University Press.

Mechanic, D. (1996). Changing medical organization and the erosion of trust. *Milbank Quarterly, 74*(2), 171–89.

Mechanic, D., & Rosenthal, M. (1999). Responses of HMO medical directors to trust building in managed care. *Milbank Quarterly, 77*(3), 283–303.

Pellegrino, E. (1986). Rationing health care: The ethics of medical gatekeeping. *Journal of Contemporary Health Law Policy, 2,* 23–45.

118   *Care of the Sufferer*

Pelligrino, E. (1991). Trust and distrust in professional ethics. In E. Pelligrino, et al. (Eds.). *Ethics, trust and the professions* (pp. 68–85). Washington, D.C.: Georgetown University Press.

Pellegrino, E. (1997). Managed care at the bedside: How do we look in the moral mirror? *Kennedy Institute of Ethics Journal, 7*(4), 321–30.

Ruskin, A. (1997). Capitation: The legal implications of using capitation to affect physician decision-making processes. *Journal of Contemporary Health Law and Policy, 12,* 391–421.

Rusnak, R., et al. (1994). Misdiagnosis of acute appendicitis: Common features discovered in cases after litigation. *American Journal of Emergency Medicine, 12*(4), 397–402.

Schulmeister, L. (1999). Chemotherapy medication errors: Descriptions, severity and contributing factors. *Oncology Nursing Forum, 26*(6), 1033–42.

Seligman, A. (2000). Trust, confidence and the problem of civility. In L. Rouner (Ed.). *Civility* (pp. 65–77). Notre Dame, Ind.: University of Notre Dame Press.

Sprung, C., et al. (1997). Is the patient's right to die evolving into a duty to die? Medical decision making and ethical evaluations in health care. *Journal of Evaluation in Clinical Practice, 3*(1), 69–75.

Sulmasy, D. (1995). Managed care and managed death. *Archives of Internal Medicine, 155,* 133–36.

Thomas, C. (1997). *Taber's encyclopedic medical dictionary.* Philadelphia: F.A. Davis.

Veach, R. (1991). Allocating health resources ethically: New roles for administrators and clinicians. *Frontiers of Health Services Management, 8,*(1) 3–29.

Vezeau, T. (1997). Quality of care and critical pathways: Brave new world? *International Journal of Caring Sciences, 1*(2), 11–15.

Wear, S. (1993). *Informed consent: Patient autonomy and physician beneficence within clinical medicine.* Boston: Kluwer Academic Publishers.

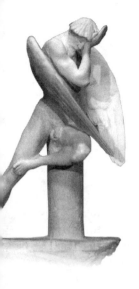

Chapter 8

How Can the Characteristics of Individual Suffering Be Elicited?

While suffering may be unavoidable, hardening the
heart to the cry of suffering is a human act.
AARON SINGER (1969, P. 50)

Chapter 2 presented the model of suffering with its components of
isolation, hopelessness, vulnerability, loss, and fear. Those themes
were explored through literary depictions in Chapter 3 to enhance
clinicians' sensitivity to their expression. Chapter 6 addressed the
prevention of suffering in relation to the identified commonalities of
the model of suffering. In this chapter, specific strategies are offered so
that health-care professionals can enhance attention to suffering in
their practices.

Witnessing suffering is inherently a formidable task because it
causes health professionals to confront their own mortality. It
challenges clinicians to abandon their familiar and comfortable
scientific perspective and to tolerate a measure of uncertainty—an
ability required to comprehend the world of the sufferer (Pozatek,
1994). To address a particular patient's suffering, one must ordinarily
ask the patient about it because "So many hurting people in the world
never call for help" (Willig, 2001, p. 15). Indeed, the patient often
lacks descriptive language. Egendorf (1995) has described suffering
patients as feeling that " . . . some nameless, unspeakable nothing
clutches at them, demanding a response that they do not know how to
give" (p. 20). Even though voicing suffering is difficult for many
patients, Egendorf defines the responsibility of clinicians to ". . . bear
with the other while he or she struggles to say what so far has been
inexpressible" (p. 11). This conundrum requires attention to some
details of the interaction between the sufferer and the health-care
professional.

Particularizing Suffering

> The single individual who, in distress, in suffering is looking for help
> and submits to medical treatment (or is entrusted to the care of a
> physician) can never, or only in rare exceptional cases, be
> comprehended in a way which the totality and singularity of his
> being would demand. Dismayed by our incapacity to meet the
> individual as a primal entity . . . we dare, nevertheless, not to
> despair or withdraw in resignation (*Philosophy of Karl Jaspers*).
> K. KOLLE (1981, P. 463)

The above quote encapsulates the difficulty of discovering the nature
and extent of a patient's suffering. Questions such as "What is this
illness like for you?" encourage dialogue that assists the clinician to
identify the patient's perception of his or her current situation.
Sometimes patients themselves will seek help and initiate
communication by asking, "Why did this happen?" There is no
simple answer to this question, for many factors contribute to the
picture of suffering that clinicians observe; however, identifying the
individual's unique experience is of primary importance. Even
cultural characteristics can be reductionistic unless health-care
professionals attend to individual meanings (Kleinman, 1991).
Although some responses are suggested in the following discussion,
most experienced professionals possess the needed personal,
counseling, and clinical skills to help patients after a clear picture of
the suffering emerges.

ALONENESS

The wisdom of the healers of old, who regarded the restoration of
relationships as essential to healing, has been generally lost (Katon &
Sullivan, 1997). Arguably, the conventions of modern health-care
practice often exclude and depersonalize patients and thereby make
them feel alone in their predicament of illness. Although distress and
pain typically bring patients to health-care professionals, attention to
their suffering is often excluded from consideration, as verified by an
analysis of taped medical consultations (Heath, 1989). This process
may achieve correct diagnoses and treatments, but it engenders
aloneness. The poet Coleridge (1798/1912) described well the essence
of agonizing loneliness when he wrote of the ancient mariner, "So
lonely 'twas that God himself scarce seemed to be" (Part VII, lines
599–600). Behaviorally, some patients may react to their undesired
separateness by appearing to be passive or withdrawn. Others may

express anger at feeling abandoned in their distress. On occasion, patients use physical symptoms to seek human caring (Katon & Sullivan, 1997), a process that may ultimately be frustrating for them and for health-care professionals from whom they often seek attention.

The antidote for aloneness is connectedness. To assess the degree of patient aloneness, the health-care professional may ask, *"How do people who are important in your life see your illness or disability?"* With this question, health-care professionals often discover what people central in the patient's life believe about the illness, treatment, and care provided. The views of significant others may be a source of distress or support to the patient. Some patients have strong bonds of family and friendship that remain unchanged and may be sufficiently nurturing during illness to negate their aloneness. In other cases, however, it is the illness that alters those relationships and disrupts bonds that patients have regarded as both normal and enduring. Therefore, the clinician may ask, *"What personal problems have been caused by your illness?"* For example, when the head of a household becomes ill, practical problems related to finances and child care arise. In addition, control must be relinquished to others, and consequently the roles, responsibilities, feelings, and relationships of other family members may be altered dramatically. Often family members and support persons become distressed by caregiving, particularly if they are over involved. According to Coyne, et al. (1988), as family caregiving responsibilities become taxing and extended, the strain becomes apparent to patients who become more stoic. The patient's self-control then may make the helpers doubt the severity of the illness, resulting in unfavorably altered relationships. Family and friends may even withdraw, thus causing patients to feel even more alone because they lack someone who enters into their world and cares for their singularity.

A follow-up question that may be asked is, *"Whom can you rely on and trust?"* Even one loving family member or friend can penetrate the solitude if a good relationship existed prior to the illness. When such a person (or persons) is available, the health-care professional is adjunctive to the primary support person; however, clinicians need to be alert to a caregiver's fatigue and offer such assistance as may be available. Sometimes patients literally have neither family nor friends, and health-care professionals become support persons temporarily. In the meantime, new social support systems, often triggered by the clinician, can be brought into place by social workers, religious or community organizations, and sometimes paid helpers.

HOPELESSNESS

Hopelessness, too, is an unwanted companion to suffering. Health-care professionals sometimes contribute to the hopelessness by their detached manner. In *The Wall* (Sartre, 1948), three prisoners in a seemingly desperate situation await execution the next morning. With them is a compassionless physician who has been assigned to observe them. During the night, Ibbieta, one of the condemned, reflects that the physician ". . . wasn't interested in what we thought; he came to watch our bodies, bodies dying in agony while yet alive" (p. 20).

For some patients, hopelessness may be the most visible characteristic of their suffering because they believe that they are in an unchosen situation where nothing will afford relief. They may respond with resignation, anxiety, anger, or guilt (Budd, 1993). Farran, et al. (1995) further describes the condition of hopelessness:

> Hopelessness constitutes an essential experience of the human condition. It functions as a feeling of despair and discouragement; a thought process that expects nothing; and a behavioral process in which the person attempts little or takes inappropriate action (p. 25).

In fact, for the philosopher Kierkegaard (1954), "The ultimate suffering is despair" (p. 150). Encountering a patient who feels disconsolate often reveals a person who has abandoned his goals or at least feels them to be threatened or unreachable. To provide comfort it becomes incumbent on the clinician to discover what the patient's hopes were by asking, *"Before this illness/disability, what were your expectations or plans for the months/years ahead?"* In general, the magnitude of suffering will be proportional to the extent to which patients are, or perceive themselves to be, unable to attain valued goals and perform related activities. Distress, shock, and depression may be expected as patients relinquish cherished goals. As indicated earlier, clinically significant depression, which may be evidenced as eating and sleeping disorders or suicide threats or attempts, needs to be identified by the generalist and the patient referred to mental health professionals for treatment. Some patients, therefore, should be asked, *"Do you ever feel like just giving up?"* to further evaluate the need for consultation with a mental health professional and to assess the urgency of that need. Hopelessness and depression may be related to the illness or disability itself or to the failure of attempts to resolve some of the problems associated with the disorder.

Initially, hopelessness may be addressed by focusing the patient's attention on more manageable situations or a shorter time frame.

Clinicians may ask, *"What hopes do you have for today and tomorrow?"* This question elicits the patient's perception of his or her health status and perhaps, more important, functional status. The realities of some illnesses dictate that the achievement of certain long-term goals is no longer feasible. The terminally ill patient, for example, is forced to relinquish career and family goals and, indeed, her own being and the future itself. What can she hope for? The patient can hope for something today that health-care professionals are in a position to furnish; that is, symptomatic relief and attentive caring. Obviously too, the alleviation of much suffering can be achieved by caring for pathological pain, vomiting, dyspnea, cough, or other physical symptoms (Chapman & Garvin, 1993).

Additionally, other kinds of distress require both physical and empathic attention by the clinician. Among dying patients, for example, the health-care professional might facilitate contact with family and friends, provide opportunities for them to be involved in decisions about care, and attend scrupulously to their cleanliness, comfort, and appearance. Thus, by their actions, clinicians can help patients achieve what Blum (1985) has called expectant faith. Even those who appear to have nothing to hope for can have their expectations fulfilled each day by clinicians who furnish consistent symptom control as well as competent, detailed, and personal care.

For those with physical impairments, some suffering may be alleviated by employing restorative therapies, using assistive devices, or providing helpers. Such strategies not only reinstate function, at least in part, but also restore confidence and serve to re-establish patients' connections with the world. Rehabilitation, for example, facilitates achievement of some goals that make possible the restoration of patients' social roles such as those of parent, spouse, or employee (Rawleson, 1986). Without such attention, patients may perceive their bodies to be disintegrating and feel powerless to change the situation, thereby sustaining feelings of hopelessness. Sometimes support groups are of value because the participants, having experienced a similar challenge, are both credible and helpful.

In summary, the health-care professional's role is to manage the illness or disability competently, perceive the extent and nature of the patient's sense of hopelessness, and link patients to appropriate services. Hopelessness is a disabling characteristic of suffering because, as the ancient Israelites observed, "When hope is crushed, the heart is crushed . . ." (Proverbs 13:12). When hope exists, however, its presence may be calming or energizing.

VULNERABILITY

In illnesses, particularly those with a sudden onset or a prolonged and unpredictable course, many patients suffer because they feel that they are increasingly susceptible to further harm; thus, they feel vulnerable. Health-care professionals often are predisposed to address vulnerability from the perspective of factual information only and fail to perceive patients' emotional distress. Their anxiety and fears may even be deemed unrealistic. Yet, Montaigne in his *Essays* (1580) elucidated the significance of fear that is entangled with vulnerability:

> The thing in the world I am most afraid of is fear. It exceeds in sharpness all other disturbances. . ... And the many people who, unable to endure the pangs of fear, have hanged or drowned themselves, or dashed themselves from a precipice, have sufficiently taught us that fear is more important and unsupportable than death itself
>
> ZEITLIN (1934, P. 62).

Fear

Clinically, fear is often most evident in patients' expressions of vulnerability because those who are fear-filled perceive themselves to be powerless to deal with the situation that threatens them. In a study of patients' and professionals' perceptions of suffering, Lindholm & Erikson (1993) conclude that "The inner obstacle (in suffering) is fear of powers beyond one's own control . . ." (p. 1356). The authors alert clinicians that such fear and suffering is expressed according to the individual personality of the patient. Emotional expressions may include a variety of personality types, including but not limited to ". . . the silent patient, the direct, the aggressive, the isolated, the defensive, the doubter, the selfish, the symbolizer, the actor and the non-verbal" (pp. 1357–58). Consequently, some patients who express suffering through these behaviors may be judged as difficult, not suffering!

Fear is the progenitor of suffering and as such mandates attention. It evokes a sense of vulnerability and powerlessness that is uniquely constructed from individual, subjective experience. It is prudent, therefore, to ask patients who are suffering, *"What would make you feel safer?"* In answering this question, patients often name their greatest fear. Their reply may indicate an underlying desire for more information or greater autonomy, or simply for the presence of a supportive person. Lack of information results in uncertainty, anxiety, and increased vulnerability because patients often fill their knowledge gaps with inaccuracies, some of which are quite frightening to them.

Reducing vulnerability requires accurate information offered in language that patients can understand, and at a time when symptoms are minimal and they can listen.

Good communication honors the patient as a human being by virtue of the clinician's time and attention, and it reduces uncertainty. One study of cancer patients' perceptions of beneficial professional behaviors found that 38 percent of the respondents regarded the provision of medical information as a helpful physician behavior, whereas just 27 percent of the patients reported technically competent care as useful (Dakof & Taylor, 1990). These findings suggest that health-care professionals have different priorities from patients and that clinicians may not appreciate how difficult it is for patients to negotiate the health-care system and obtain factual and complete information about their illness, its treatment, and its consequences. Asking *"Do you need more information about any aspect of your illness or care?"* helps to reduce this disparity of power and perspective and to validate the patient's role in the management of his or her illness.

Pain

Although fear may exist independently of pain, it almost always accompanies it and engenders a sense of vulnerability. It is critical, therefore, to ask the patient, *"How much unrelieved pain do you have?"* because pain engenders a sense of defenselessness and initiates beliefs such as, "My body is being destroyed by pain." Pain makes patients fearful and vulnerable when they must depend on others for its relief. When pain extends endlessly into the future, it becomes suffering. Asking *"What does or does not relieve your pain?"* validates the pain and guides care. Failure to correctly evaluate and alleviate pain when it is possible to do so is morally reprehensible.

Control

Patients' levels of vulnerability and needs to influence their care may be further determined by a question such as, *"How could your situation be improved?"* Patients may set forth ideas that are implemented easily, such as requests for dietary changes or for more rest. Offering patients more opportunities to make decisions about their care, when possible, can reduce their vulnerability and afford them a sense of added control. For example, a patient with extensive burns may be invited to decide when dressing changes that involve pain, in spite of premedication, will be performed. Other strategies such as employing distraction techniques or relaxation exercises may also enable patients to feel more autonomous, less vulnerable, and perhaps better able to tolerate their suffering. In still other situations, patients may feel that they are partners in achieving control if they have adequate assistance with their activities or health problems. For instance, persons with loss of mobility feel vulnerable to falls and further injury when lifted or moved by unskilled personnel. Brief training of staff by physical therapists, professional nurses, or others can develop better transfer techniques that will benefit both patients and staff. Such attention to detail generally reduces the patient's sense of vulnerability and improves her quality of life and well-being.

Less concretely, but equally important, patients also feel vulnerable because they lose the mastery that they had over their lives when they were healthy. Hospitalization, in fact, requires them to be dependent and sometimes to be apart from those persons and groups who offer support. For example, the newlywed with a sudden severe cardiac impairment is forced to modify his role as husband, abandon his belief in youthful good health, and confront his threatened status as a wage earner. Altered social roles, together with fear, pain, and diminished control, evoke a sense of vulnerability when the body is impaired. When patients sense that they are overwhelmed, subsequent feelings of vulnerability, powerlessness, and dread ensue. Health-care professionals must identify and seek to support the healing of these wounds.

LOSS

Illness alters how patients see their world and tests their purposes and values. At the very least, patients lose connection with their usual life patterns and become self-absorbed and preoccupied with their symptoms, their treatment, and the potential outcome of their condition. In illnesses that are serious or perceived to be serious, patients often begin to pose significant questions about themselves and their world. Especially in serious illness, patients ask, "What is the purpose of my existence?" and "Why must I suffer?" Precipitated by awareness that they have had a significant loss, many patients struggle to bring understanding and reason to their suffering, challenging long-held views and values. Their loss may be the deprivation of good health; limited mobility; loss of an opportunity, skill, or career; or even the impending loss of life itself.

Altered Meanings

As patients become conscious of their losses, or in some cases anticipate them, suffering ensues. Sometimes patients will communicate their deprivation and suffering by saying, "What's to become of me?" or "What does this all mean?" These are questions about the nature of their existence, rather than requests for information. Astute clinicians sense this struggle and invite dialogue by saying something like, *"Has your illness made you question what is important?"* In patients' responses, health-care professionals may detect patients' needs to grapple with the nature and personal significance of their suffering, which may seem overpowering. Indeed, Mason (1977) has defined suffering as the experience ". . . of being acted on, and of being changed from a former state in a way that is inconsistent with its (the individual's) present sense of well-being" (p. 95). Frequently significant illness destroys one's very identity and personhood.

As patients endeavor to make sense of the havoc in their lives, they may seek or call on philosophical or religious views to interpret the meaning of their losses and subsequent suffering. Others develop their own truths that may be individually satisfying. Some of the common interpretations of suffering identified by Foley (1988) include punishment, testing, bad luck, submission to the laws of nature, resignation to the will of God, acceptance of the human condition, personal growth, defensiveness, minimizing, and divine or redemptive perspectives (pp. 321–28). If patients are unaware of their interpretations, their suffering may seem meaningless (Blocker, 1974). When patients are aware of the significance they have accorded their suffering, clinicians may simply acknowledge it, occasionally validate interpretations, and at times identify resources. As Tedeschi, et al. (1998) have written, some patients ". . . experience further spiritual development [as a result of trauma]." They have ". . . a greater sense of somehow being connected to something transcendent, in ways that were not possible before the struggle with trauma" (p. 14).

Specific life situations or consequences of clinical problems that produce suffering may be elicited by a question such as, *"What is at stake for you?"* Here factual clinical information may be helpful in giving hope to patients who inappropriately expect a more negative illness outcome than the facts predict. They may be reassured by learning that improvement can be made over time, that loss of social or occupational participation due to disabling symptoms can be restored or modified, or that loss of function can be improved, if only in part, by rehabilitation or assistive devices. Much information in the health-care literature contributes to meeting a patient's needs for practical assistance.

Answers to *"What is at stake?"* often reveal how patients see their world—miserable, abhorrent, or hopeful, or it may also reveal more complex human problems. For example, an in-depth study of 14 patients with rheumatoid arthritis revealed their perception that they had disintegrated as persons and that their pain and anguish had resulted in a "shattered self" (Dildy, 1996). Somehow, most of these patients were able to "reconstruct" themselves. Such positive reorientation often requires that values and meanings be identified and reviewed; then possibly modified, changed, or affirmed by patients. Byock (1994) states the matter succinctly. He writes that sufferers found relief when they ". . . surrendered *who they were* to a new reality of *who they are* . . . . Often patients report an experienced sense of connection to a timeless, enduring construct" (p. 13).

Endurance

Most challenging for the clinician is the proper course of support for the patient who suffers greatly, either with unrelieved symptoms, spiritual distress, or an unacceptable quality of life. Ultimately, what is at risk for some of those who are in true agony is the choice between continued endurance and suicide or requests for euthanasia. Much information may be found in the health-care literature concerning suicide and requests for euthanasia, particularly when patients are in torment after palliative care has been only partially successful.

Less is known about what constitutes and supports endurance. Endurance of some patients fails when they face a dreadful future. They appear to just "give up." Yet other patients, in seemingly similar circumstances, endure their suffering and sometimes develop comforting insights. Morse & Carter (1996) have set forth the intriguing idea that patients in physiological jeopardy enter a state that the authors call "enduring to survive." Patients may "endure to live" when their situations are more tolerable. Only when patients have more resilience, they postulate, is suffering and the attendant emotion initiated. In such circumstances, patients may be assisted to identify helpful alternatives. Asking *"How did you get through other difficult times in your life?"* not only assists patients to retain their identity as decision makers, but also draws on their experiences with previous stress and trauma. Sometimes, patients describe a strong family member, public figure, friend, or ancestor who prevailed over difficulty and who becomes a role model or a mentor in their suffering. When patients have had successful experiences with other stressful situations, they may cope better in similar or even different circumstances (Garber, 1980).

Responses to these questions alert health-care professionals that patients endure losses in different ways. To assume that the "correct way" to experience loss is to follow a prescribed pattern often leads to inappropriate care, lacking in emotional support. For instance, Wortman & Silver (1989) found that empirical evidence refuted the widely held belief that depression and distress are inevitable consequences of loss. Other myths that were *not* supported in their research include the beliefs that later problems are an inevitable consequence of little expression of distress, delayed resolution of loss causes eventual problems, and coping with significant loss requires prolonged resolution. In these and other characteristics of individual suffering, Erickson's well stated maxim guides the clinician, ". . . every human being's suffering is unique and bears the sufferer's name" (Graneheim, et al., 1997, p. 146).

When asked, *"What is most frightening (or of greatest concern) for you?"* the patient's fears are elicited and can be addressed. For instance, patients who become ill in a culture unlike their own or who have had little acquaintance with the health-care system, experience fear and anxiety related to the unfamiliar. Other fears patients have may be related to a specific medical procedure or an illness outcome. Seriously ill patients who do not have an immediate clinical concern may reveal that their greatest fear is loss of an acceptable quality of life or loss of their own existence. The circumstances that precipitate fear often cannot be changed, but patients can sometimes develop other ways of perceiving a situation. In addition, the stated dread may alter care priorities and guide changes in care to modify the fear. Sometimes, merely asking about the patients' greatest concerns is comforting because it allows them to emerge from anonymity and affirms the humanity that they share with clinicians.

Impending Death

For most people, the ultimate loss is terminal illness and death. Although humans have the unique capacity to contemplate their own deaths and some face death without fear, others deny its inevitability. "Every day we are dying and in the process of change, and yet we think we will go on forever," writes Saint Jerome in the first century (Scourfield, 1993, p. 73). For most patients, sustaining their life is the highest value, but patients who are able to say, "I am afraid of dying," have overcome the obstacle of denial. Typically patients make this disclosure initially to a family member, friend, or trusted religious advisor or a health-care professional who is "safe"; that is, one who is compassionate and able to sustain a relationship. If a clinician knows that the patient's fear is not validated by clinical data, then the patient may be asked, "What makes you fear that you will die?" In some cases, correct and adequate medical information will comfort the patient and relieve the fear. In other situations, the patient will require supportive care and perhaps professional counseling when death is near. Although a body of literature on the care and counseling of the dying exists for clinicians to consult, development of such end-of-life competencies is generally not included in the education of health-care generalists. Unfortunately, clergy, pastoral care staff, or other counselors sometimes work parallel to, but not with, other health-care professionals to care for the dying. With the exception of hospice and other selected settings, the lack of coordination among professionals may be related to differing perspectives, but more often it is the consequence of a health-care system that allows little time and furnishes little structure for interdisciplinary efforts on behalf of patients.

In response to the patient's expression of fear of death, a responsible clinician might ask, "What beliefs do you have?" or "What is death like for you?" Two types of patient perspectives are possible. First, the belief that death is annihilation may be expressed. The power of death and its depiction as a state lacking in sensation was described by Lamont (1990) who writes, "For if we are right in calling immortality an illusion the dead have no consciousness that they are missing life or that the living are missing them. They cannot grieve over being parted from those whom they love" (p. 267). In contrast, others share a hopeful expectation of a blissful state such as that found in Indian spiritual philosophy (Aurobindo, 1981): "From non-being to true being, from the darkness to the Light, from death to Immortality" (*The Upanishands* I.3.28, p. 419). It is important for the clinician not only to determine the particular patient perspective that is operative, but also to listen for the variations of views within a stated belief on immortality. Among these variations are the influence of natural processes, reincarnation or rebirth, resurrection of the body, and immortality of the soul.

Asking *"What sustains you now?"* is a way for health-care professionals to elicit what resources of character, spirituality, philosophy, or interpretation of previous experience patients can marshal in their struggles. As they ponder the significance and sometimes opportunities for spiritual growth, patients often affirm, discover, or create interpretations of events that are comforting. Some patients put their faith in medical science. For others, illness and suffering merely validate their belief that suffering is inherent in life or that life is capricious and ultimately futile. Others find a transcendent reality beyond their present state. But some patients are not sustained by meaningfulness, and the world of the sufferer remains incoherent and insecure. Today's patients are often ill-prepared to deal with their diseased and hurting bodies and with the brevity of life (Van den Berg, 1980). Those who have thought little about death tax clinicians' resources to the limit when meaninglessness causes extreme suffering. Sometimes suffering is so tragic that it eludes meaning. The condition of patients in these circumstances was expressed by the grieving poet Whittier (1850/1971) on the death of Daniel Webster:

> All else is gone; from those great eyes
> The soul has fled:
> When faith is lost, when honor dies,
> The man is dead! (p. 80)

When a spark of meaningfulness remains, or can be kindled, some patients find comfort in spiritual beliefs or in religious symbols or observances. Sometimes the experience of suffering itself can be healing or redemptive. In recalling past pleasures and accomplishments, if their lives heretofore have been satisfying, other patients find peace. "The past is ours, and nothing's in safer keeping than what has been" writes Seneca in a consoling letter to Lucilius in the first century (Barker, 1932, p. 175). Still other patients subscribe to Frankl's (1946/1984) assertion that meaning is inherent in life itself—in joy as well as in suffering. As a survivor of the horrors of the Holocaust, Frankl's wisdom evolved from suffering. He wrote, "One thing is never lost . . . the last of human freedoms—to choose one's attitude in any given set of circumstances, to choose one's own way" (p. 86).

For patients who do not embrace a sustaining belief structure, as for those who do, the appropriate care recommendation is the prevention of further suffering and what Donley (1991) has called "compassionate accompaniment" (p. 179). Those who suffer and do not find transcendence must neither be deprecated, blamed, nor abandoned because at times suffering is seemingly beyond meaning. Their courage is displayed by simply continuing to live in agony, as they experience the loss of life's relationships, purposes, values, and significance and the extinguishing of life itself. Health-care professionals who tolerate their own end-of-life questions and anxieties to comfort such patients display exemplary courage as well.

What Is The Suffering Like?

The following table recapitulates this chapter. The key questions identified furnish a guide for particularizing suffering within the context of the model of suffering (Table 8–1) that includes the symptoms, beliefs, and endangered values associated with suffering. The table is a guide for clinician-patient interactions and may be especially useful to health-care professionals who have recently resolved to systematically incorporate the care of suffering into their practices. The table can inform clinicians and give direction to their practices, but it should *never* be employed as a data collection instrument.

SUMMARY

In illness, suffering exists in a dimension that differs from organic disease. Clinicians need to be intentional to discover the characteristics of a patient's suffering because the origins and nature of it determine the care required. Merely recognizing that the characteristics of suffering exist does not alone produce understanding of a particular patient's experience. By assessing suffering, health-care professionals affirm patients' abilities to understand and report their experiences and validate their capacities for self-determination. Certain key questions can elicit the essence and nature of individual suffering for the clinician and can guide patients as they articulate their interpretation of it. This mutuality provides a basis for resolving some of suffering's attendant problems and for enabling the patient to better accept, endure, or transcend them. Although clinicians may be active in symptom management and in cure, they often and importantly are also a sustaining presence from whom patients can borrow strength. Correct care delivered with compassion is the highest calling of the true health-care professional.

PRECEPT FOR PRACTICE

Health-care professionals may choose to fashion compassionate care within the life view of patients and thereby accompany them in the human reality of suffering.

TABLE 8–1. Eliciting The Characteristics of Individual Suffering

Observable Symptoms	Underlying Belief	Key Questions	Substance: Endangered Values
Changed relationships with others Solitary Unsupported Separated Abandoned	I am alone.	How do people who are important in your life see your illness/disability? What personal problems have been caused by this illness? Whom can you rely on and trust?	Being cared about for one's own sake is good. The ability to care about and for others is good.
Altered expectations Discouraged Ineffective Oppressed Despairing	I am without hope.	Before this illness/disability, what were your expectations of the months/years ahead? Do you ever feel like just giving up? What hopes do you have for today and tomorrow?	Having acceptable alternatives is good.
Damaging pain, discomfort, and/or distress Unease Intimidated Endangered Full of dread	I am vulnerable.	What would make you feel safer? Do you need more information concerning any aspect of your Illness or care? How much unrelieved pain do you have? What does/does not relieve your pain? How could your situation be improved?	The absence of pain and distress is good. The full use of one's abilities is good.
Lack of coherence Disadvantaged Deprived Ruined Without meaning	I have experienced (or will experience) a great loss.	Has your illness made you question what is important? What is at stake for you? How did you get through other difficult times in your life? What is most frightening for you? (Or of greatest concern?) What sustains you now?	Having satisfying beliefs about one's place in the world is good. It is good to exist.

REFERENCES

Aurobindo, S. (1981). *The Upanishands, Part One.* Mt. Tremper, NY: Matagiri, Distributor.

Barker, E. (trans.). (First Century/1932). *Seneca's Letters to Lucilius, Volume II.* Oxford: at the Clarendon Press.

Blocker, G. (1974). *The meaning of meaninglessness.* The Hague: Martinus Nijoff.

Blum, L. (1985). Beyond medicine: Healing power in the doctor-patient relationship. *Psychological Reports, 57,* 399–427.

Budd, M. (1993). Human suffering: Road to illness or gateway to learning? *Advances: The Journal of Mind-Body Health, 9*(3), 28–35.

Byock, I. (1994). When suffering persists . . .. *Journal of Palliative Care, 10*(2), 8–13.

Chapman, C., & Garvin, J. (1993). Suffering and its relationship to pain. *Journal of Palliative Care, 9*(2), 5–13.

Coleridge, S. (1798/1912). The rime of the ancient mariner. In E.H. Coleridge (Ed.). *The complete poetical works of Samuel Taylor Coleridge,* (pp. 187–209). Oxford: at the Clarendon Press.

Coyne, J., et al. (1988). Chapter 11, The other side of support. In B. Gottlieb (Ed.). *Marshalling Social Support.* (pp. 305–30). Newbury Park, Calif.: Sage Publications.

Dakof, G., & Taylor, S. (1990). Victim's perceptions of social support: What is helpful from whom? *Journal of Personality and Social Psychology, 58*(1), 80–89.

Dildy, S. (1996). Suffering in people with rheumatoid arthritis. *Applied Nursing Research, 9*(4), 177–83.

Donley, R. (1991). Spiritual dimensions of health care: Nursing's mission. *Nursing and Health Care, 12*(4), 178–83.

Egendorf, A. (1995). Hearing people through their pain. *Journal of Traumatic Stress, 8*(1), 5–28.

Farran, C., et al. (1995). *Hope and hopelessness: Critical clinical constructs.* Thousand Oaks, Calif.: Sage Publications.

Foley, D. (1988). 11 interpretations of personal suffering. *Journal of Religion and Health, 27*(4), 321–28.

Frankl, V. (1946/1984). *Man's search for meaning.* New York: Washington Square Press.

Garber, J. (1980). *Human Helplessness.* New York: Academic Press.

Goldberg, C. (1986). Concerning human suffering. Weekly scientific meeting, Ottawa General Hospital. *Psychiatric Journal of the University of Ottawa, 11*(2), 97–104.

Good News Bible (1992). New York: American Bible Society.

Graneheim, U., et al. (1997). *Scandinavian Journal of Caring Science, 11*(3), 145–50.

Heath, C. (1989). Pain talk: The expression of suffering in the medical consultation. *Social Psychology Quarterly, 52*(2), 113–25.

Katon, W., & Sullivan, M.(1997). Of healing and human suffering. *Journal of the American Board of Family Practice, 10*(1), 62–65.

Kierkegaard, S. (1954). *Fear and trembling: The sickness unto death.* Garden City, NJ: Doubleday.

Kleinman, R. (1991). Suffering and its professional transformations: Toward an ethnography of interpersonal experience. *Journal of Culture, Medicine and Psychiatry, 15*(3), 275–301.

Kolle, K. (1981). Karl Jaspers as psychotherapist. In P. Schlipp (Ed.). *The philosophy of Karl Jaspers.* (pp. 437–66). LaSalle, Ill.: Open Court Publishing.

Lamont, C. (1990). *The illusion of immortality.* New York: Half Moon Foundation.

Lindholm, L., & Erickson, K. (1993). To understand and alleviate suffering in a caring culture. *Journal of Advanced Nursing, 18,* 1354–61.

Mason, D. (1977). Some abstract, yet crucial thoughts about suffering. *Dialogue, 16,* 91–100.

Morse, J., & Carter, B. (1996). The essence of enduring and expressions of suffering: The reformulation of self. *Scholarly Inquiry for Nursing Practice: An International Journal, 10*(1), 43–60.

Pozatek, E. (1994). The problem of certainty: Clinical social work in the postmodern era. *Social Work, 39*(4), 396–403.

Rawleson, M. (1986). The sense of suffering. *The Journal of Medicine and Philosophy, 11*(1), 39–62.

Sartre, J. (1948). The wall. In *Intimacy and other stories.* (L. Alexander, trans.). (pp. 7–38). New York: A New Directions Book.

Scourfield, J. (1993). *Consoling Heliodorus: A commentary on Jerome, Letter, 60.* Oxford: Clarendon Press.

Singer, A. (1989). Human responses to suffering in Rabbinic teaching. *Dialogue and Alliance, 3,* 49–57.

Tedeschi, R., et al. (Eds.). (1998). *Post-traumatic growth: Positive Change in the Aftermath of Crisis.* Mahwah, NJ: Lawrence Erlbaum Associates.

Van den Berg. (1980). *The psychology of the sickbed.* New York: Humanities Press.

Whittier, J.G. (1850/1971). Ichabod. In R.P. Warren (Ed.). *John Greenleaf Whittier's Poetry.* (pp. 79–80). Minneapolis: The University of Minnesota Press.

Willig, J. (2001). *Lessons from the school of suffering.* Cincinnati, Ohio: St. Anthony Messenger Press.

Wortman, C., & Silver, R. (1989). The myths of coping with loss. *Journal of Consulting and Clinical Psychology, 57*(3), 349–57.

Zeitlin, J. (Ed./trans.). (1580/1934). *The Essays of Michel de Montaigne, Volume One.* New York: Alfred Knopf.

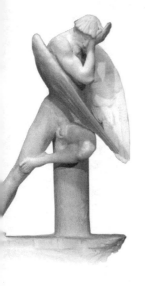

Chapter 9

Summary and Conclusion

Everyone who is born holds dual citizenship, in the kingdom of the well and in the kingdom of the sick.

S. SONTAG (1978, P. 3)

The previous chapters have attempted to clarify the nature of suffering for health-care professionals and describe some approaches to caring for sufferers. However, some health-care professionals may feel overwhelmed by the magnitude and complexity of the responsibility. Although a number of clinicians are highly effective in perceiving suffering and helping patients to endure it, others are at the beginning of their journeys to develop that level of competence. For those persons, some summary and guidance may be in order.

First, the clinician ought to be aware of forces that support denial of suffering. Popular culture in the United States holds that it is possible to avoid suffering. This optimistic belief is supported by faith in science and technology that seems to hold the promise of preventing or fully alleviating suffering. This view is diametrically opposed to that expressed by Montaigne (1580/1958) about 500 years ago: "We are born to grow old, to grow weak, to be sick, in spite of medicine" (Zeitlin, p. 835). Although science deals with most pathology successfully, it inherently neglects how patients experience their illnesses and treatments. This insight is required to care for the suffering that accompanies disease or disability.

Second, clinicians are obligated to minimize or prevent suffering, or to ameliorate it. Thoughtlessness, poorly managed physical problems, unrecognized major depressive disorders and certain characteristics of the health-care system itself lead to unnecessary suffering. Such conditions can often be relieved or eliminated by compassionate and competent care that is personalized and attentive

136

to detail and by creative applications of known treatments or illness-management modalities.

Third, health-care professionals should recognize that some aspects of suffering may not be wholly negative. Few persons would choose to suffer; however, suffering can sometimes be transforming. Some sufferers draw on philosophical or spiritual beliefs to help them endure their travails and become strengthened by their ordeals. Suffering may even be instructive and lead to new ways of being and behaving. Like Leonardo's *Adoration of the Magi,* which depicts pathology (cutaneous lesions) along with beauty (Marchetti, 1997), suffering, which appears ugly, and the beauty of the person who is the patient, can coexist.

Fourth, clinicians need to develop realistic expectations about their strengths and limitations in helping patients who are suffering. Some suffering is inevitable and cannot be eliminated; however, patients and their families sometimes naively expect clinicians to remove all suffering. Assuming that symptoms have been well managed and unnecessary physical suffering prevented, the resolution of existential suffering ultimately resides with the sufferer. He alone knows fully his past experience, present concerns, and future hopes in the context of his particularized sustaining values. Many patients do employ that information meaningfully to come to terms with their suffering. As fellow human beings, clinicians can always be attentive, sometimes provide respites or resolve specific problems, and occasionally shepherd the patient to a place of greater emotional and spiritual comfort. Often health-care professionals can only witness suffering because it exceeds their knowledge and emotional wisdom.

This work has analyzed the complex human phenomenon of suffering and has advocated that health-care professionals identify patients' human needs and provide careful, ongoing attention. In some situations, that level of care may be possible. But the realities of clinical practice in most environments where health care is provided preclude such thorough practice. In such circumstances, the choice is not between comprehensive care and no care. Rather, it is a commitment to simply do what can be done because that is the responsibility entrusted to us.

A place to begin for clinicians is to wrest 10 minutes from each hectic day to devote to one selected, suffering patient, believing that such attention will have a positive effect on the illness experience of that individual. Health-care professionals may select patients who are in agony, the most dreadful form of suffering. Patients in this state have the most desperate need for attention from a compassionate and competent clinician. In some specialties, clinicians can predict times of suffering by the course of the illness or its treatment. Situations such as sharing an unfavorable prognosis call for unfailing attention to the suffering related to that defining moment. The clinician's care in those precious moments must embrace the selected patient as if that patient were the only one needing care. Attentiveness and understanding how a patient perceives his suffering—as well as the presence of the clinician—initiate a bond that bespeaks compassion and comfort. Whenever possible, the act of caring needs to be expressed in practical ways, if only through small consoling acts that communicate human concern and penetrate the darkness of suffering.

Initially it may be uncomfortable for clinicians who decide to incorporate care of suffering into their practices, for the change is akin to developing a new habit. Begin by selecting just one relevant question from Table 8–1, "Eliciting the Characteristics of Individual Suffering". Pose that question to a selected patient and be prepared to listen, even if you cannot respond with confidence. Sometimes just listening and nodding or reflecting the content is enough to warm the area with humanity. When you are comfortable asking the first question, move on to another, and a relationship will begin to build. With experience will come confidence to integrate other strategies into patient care, wisdom born of experience, and a renewed sense of personal and professional achievement.

Finally, it is imperative for health-care professionals to be realistic about the effect of repeatedly encountering the suffering of a stranger. Caring for the suffering person is emotionally draining and, on occasion, seemingly futile. Some patients may appreciate the considerable effort that clinicians expend to help them. Others may express anger, be manipulative or seem obstinate; yet these behaviors are often manifestations of suffering. Such patients should not be abandoned, but neither should clinicians expect to relieve all suffering and its manifestations.

Why then would health-care professionals choose to risk their inner peace and experience distress by encountering suffering? For those who regard their work as a calling, even 10 minutes devoted each day to a particular sufferer can provide an altruistic perspective and be energizing in a shift that requires attention to myriad details and seemingly unending tasks.

For many clinicians, involvement in the suffering of others may also be instructive in their own life journeys. It is a reminder that they, too, must discover what they believe and value, what gives meaning to their own lives, and what they must do to develop their own spirituality. The process that begins by helping others achieve greater equanimity eventually helps clinicians achieve their own. Occasionally a boon awaits clinicians because some who suffer will furnish a glimpse of the best that humans can aspire to be as they encounter what Jaspers has called "the boundary situations of human existence" (Schrag, 1971). Suffering cannot be regarded as a "we the healer" and "they the sufferer" phenomenon. "For, in fact, sufferer and healer are interchangeable roles: now sufferer, now healer; now helper, now helped; now giver, now receiver" (Ashbrook, 1975, p. 11).

In the end, suffering remains a mystery that eludes even the most caring and wise. Yet even partial knowledge and the complexity of suffering are not reasons for inattention or inaction. Relief of suffering is usually performed imperfectly. As those devoted to the care of vulnerable human beings, we must respond to the highest calling of our respective professions by encountering suffering that would otherwise escape attention, by attempting to understand it, and by intervening to prevent or relieve it. For, "The kingdom of suffering is a democracy, and we all stand in it or alongside it with nothing but our naked humanity. All of us have the same capacity to help and that is the good news" (Yancy, 1984, p. 92).

PRECEPT FOR PRACTICE

Encountering human suffering is both a moral and professional duty.

REFERENCES

Ashbrook, J. (1975). *Responding to pain.* Valley Forge, PA: Judson Press.

Marchetti, C., & Panconesi E. (1997). Leonardo da Vince: Beauty or human suffering in the world. Notes on pathological cutaneous alterations in the 'Adoration of the Magi.' *Journal of the European Academy of Dermatology and Venereology, 8*(2), 101–11.

Schrag, O. (1971). *Existence, existenz, and transcendence: An introduction to the philosophy of Karl Jaspers.* Pittsburgh, PA: Duquesne University Press.

Sontag, S. (1978). *Illness as Metaphor.* New York: Farrar, Straus & Sons.

Yancy, P. (1984). Helping those in pain. *Leadership, 5,*(2) 90–97.

Zeitlin, J. (Ed./trans.). (1580/1934). *The essays of Michel de Montaigne, Volume One.* New York: Alfred Knopf.

Afterword

HUMAN ASPECTS OF SUFFERING

Mildred E. Newcomb, PhD,
Professor Emerita of English
Ohio Wesleyan University, Delaware, Ohio

Most, if not all, of the educational/training programs preparing people for careers in the medical profession fall within the science discipline. Literature belongs to that other discipline known as the Humanities. The Humanities study what it is that makes us human. They are humane. We call benefactors "humanitarians." These terms remind us that our essential being, what makes us different from other animals, is rooted in our extended capacity to think and feel. Our thoughts and feelings create the qualities we consider human.

They also create many of the characteristics belonging to what we call suffering. And because our thoughts and feelings are the cumulative result of our past experiences and our reactions to them, no two people experience or deal with suffering in exactly the same way. The way I relate to pain and suffering helps define me, but it may have little to do with someone else—my patient in that hospital bed, for instance. Yet, that fact does not need to render me helpless, for literature opens the doors permitting me to enter someone else's psyche and to feel their emotions and to think their thoughts.

Many poems and plays, short stories, and novels take you into the inner life of a writer or his characters to experience their feelings and share their thinking and beliefs. If you read extensively, you will come to experience vicariously any feelings of which a human being is capable, may know exactly what the various aspects of suffering feel like even though you have never gone through them yourself, and thus may come to your patients with that special brand of understanding we call *empathy.* You will also experience ways in which suffering may be transcended or sublimated.

What you learn about suffering from literature, then, adds an entirely different dimension to understanding. This knowledge is *felt* rather than thought about. It communicates not messages or lessons, but *insights,* views from the inside.

Reading literature is neither easy nor fast. Feelings—responses to what we are experiencing—are complicated, often confused, convoluted, impossible to explain in simple terms. Maybe impossible ever to explain. The event or situation being experienced is also compounded of all the accumulated bits and pieces of a person's past experiences that have eventuated in his outlook: his ideas and beliefs and attitudes.

But to "be there" vicariously, you have to learn to read differently. You must immerse yourself in the experience described; you must imagine yourself into whatever states of mind the work calls for, whether by submission to the feelings it evokes, or by following a story with full participation, or by going through a process—or all three at once. You must become the person.

Sometimes all that a literary work requires of the reader is to experience a concentrated feeling: for example, a "lyric" poem "singing" a lament of loneliness or loss. "The End of the World," by Archibald MacLeish (1952, p. 23), comes close to being such an expression of feelings associated with suffering. Imagining yourself into this poem, you are suddenly projected into a situation familiar to most of us, for you are sitting in the bleachers of a circus tent surrounded by other spectators engrossed like you in the marvelous activities going on in its three rings. Although strange and wonderful things happen here, the world in which they take place—the safe, well-lighted, enclosed world of the "big top" is snug and secure. Then, without warning the top blows off, leaving performers and spectators exposed to a black, infinite space without form or dimensions.

How does this make you feel? If you have entered the fictive world without reservations so that the poem can work on you, what you momentarily feel when the top blows off almost exactly duplicates feelings characteristic of suffering: an amalgam of isolated abandonment, hopelessness, vulnerability, loss.

The momentary experience over, you can now think about it. MacLeish titled his poem "The End of the World." It is not about a circus at all. The poet has used the circus to provide insights into a totally different experience: what it feels like to have the "top" blow off your previously secure world. This poem can thus apply to any situation that feels like the end of the world, such as incapacitating injury or illness. It most definitely, then, may apply to your patient/sufferer whose world has narrowed into that hospital bed. If you are sensitive to what you have read, you will have immediate useful insights into the probable feelings he or she is experiencing.

Maybe your response to the poem comes not from discovery of something you have never experienced, but rather from recognition of feelings you very well know from your own experience. To see those feelings expressed can provide a kind of satisfaction for both writer and reader. ("What oft was thought but ne'er so well express'd," wrote one poet, Alexander Pope.) (1711/1951, p. 40). It can even ease the feelings brought about by suffering by enabling the sufferer, whether writer or character, to "get a handle on it." It is well understood that the need to express feelings can be the driving force behind literary, as well as, other artistic creation.

Lyrical poems represent only a small portion of literary production. More often, lyrical expression will work its way into more elaborate explorations, telling a story or following a process—for example, in "The Leg," by Karl Shapiro (1968, p. 82). This poem projects you into an event (the speaker's leg has just been amputated), and follows his thinking (a process) to a conclusion that enables him to transcend the pain and potential suffering. At first, as he struggles his way out of the anesthetic, he experiences only sensations of pain and touch and smell. Soon he begins to explore his sense of loss, which he quickly transfers from himself to the leg. He has not lost it: it has lost him. He develops a "sense of humor" about it: that is, he stands away from it with some perspective. Now he prays for the abandoned leg, which, being physical, will die. Eventually he moves into the belief that he himself is still intact. This leads him to contemplate how much of his physical body he could "lose" without being lessened as a human being. Finally, he feels joy and serenity as he decides "he" (his essential spirit) would remain even if his entire body should be lost—"hurl(ed) to the shark" (p. 82). He has successfully bypassed the suffering that could have resulted from his loss. The answer to his problem has been found in his religious faith, a most powerful force enabling the believer to sublimate even the pain and suffering surrounding death.

As a matter of fact, much of the greatest literature—at least of the Western world—circles about the "problem" of suffering and its alleviation by some kind of faith. It is, for example, a recurring theme in the Judeo-Christian *Bible,* as in the sufferings of Job and of Christ. Job does indeed endure the pain of boils and other indignities visited on him, but the source of his suffering lies in his mind as he questions why a just God would permit these pains to happen. Christ, in the Garden of Gethsemane, wrestles with the coming pain he must endure on the cross, but his suffering, too, arises from that question in his mind: *Why?*

For both Job and Christ, suffering becomes a test of faith. Other men, in Job's situation, would "curse God and die." But Job submits himself to God's will, and his suffering subsides. Christ, similarly, puts his fate in the hands of a God he trusts and faces his ordeal with serenity. Both of these accounts in the *Bible,* like lyrical poems in a play, take the reader into the experience of the sufferer to create insights. Religious faith becomes a way of transcending suffering.

These ancient stories still speak to us. The story of Job is retold in modern terms by Archibald MacLeish (1956) in his play about J.B., who agonizes over the conundrum: "If God is God, he is not good" (p. 11). That is, a "good" God would not permit pain and suffering. On the other hand, "If God is good, he is not God" (p. 11). That is, even though good, if He lacks the power to prevent pain, He is not omnipotent. Again, the answer lies in religious faith, submitting to the will of a God who can never be understood by human standards of what is fair.

It is important to remember, however, that what one person firmly believes, another may passionately reject. Religious faith is not available to everybody. Thomas Hardy, for example, in his little poem "Hap" (1976, p. 9), longs for *any* understandable sign of significance in his suffering. If he could believe that some more powerful intelligence had willed it, then he could meaningfully defy that power. In short, when any logical reason can be found for suffering (an answer to *why?*), then the suffering can be transcended. What flows from the poem "Hap," however, is the abandonment, despair, meaninglessness, and futility felt by a speaker who believes everything happens by pure chance rather than by design. The result is paralysis because any action is pointless.

A considerable body of mid-20th century literature, influenced by the movement called Existentialism, reflects this same sense of universal meaninglessness and paralysis, as in so-called "absurd" plays like *Waiting for Godot* (Beckett, 1954). In this play, the very first words of the play set up its central theme: "Nothing to be done," says Estragon (p. 7). This idea pervades the entire tragicomedy. In the last two lines, Vladimir says, "Well? Shall we go?" "Yes," Estragon replies, "Let's go." But, *"they do not move,"* (p. 61). With "Nothing to be done," any movement is pointless. This play is tragic if we are the characters involved. It is comic if we have perspective to see how absurd they are.

When *Waiting for Godot* first appeared in theaters, fascinated audiences had no idea what to make of the play. Although moved, they were totally unprepared for a play without action. But an enthralled audience of convicts viewing the play in Alcatraz, the federal prison from which no one ever escaped, knew exactly what it was about and had no difficulty whatever understanding it. They knew precisely how it felt to be one of the characters in the play for they were in a similarly meaningless existence: isolated, powerless, abandoned, and paralyzed. They were all "waiting for Godot," for something (sometimes interpreted as *God*) to appear to give their lives meaning and purpose. Yet, a general response of the audience was laughter, probably because the play enabled them to gain some perspective on their situation, recognize its absurdity, and thereby feel superior to it even if they couldn't change it. (Similar stories came out of Germany during World War II of "black humor" circulated among helpless citizens: jokes enabling them to laugh at their Nazi oppressors and thus establish a kind of superiority over them.)

In an existential world that has lost religious faith, there can be no meaning in our lives and actions beyond what we can create out of our own interpretation of our own existence. Albert Camus is a writer who explored this possibility. Camus takes Hardy one step further, declaring that meaning can come from personally defying cosmic meaninglessness. As long as I am myself alive and fighting, this belief asserts, meaning exists. Camus used the *Myth of Sisyphus* (1991) to show how such defiance is itself a way of rising above suffering, testing not our faith but our humanity. In this myth, Sisyphus spends each day toiling up a steep hill, pushing a heavy boulder ahead of him. When he reaches the top and releases the stone, it rolls once more to the bottom of the hill. It is all to do over again the next day. The dignity, even nobility, of Sysiphus, his worth as a human being, are demonstrated by the way he perseveres against impossible odds. His is the stance of all "tragic heroes," doomed but standing up bravely to face their fates in such fashion that we feel proud to share their humanity.

Another avenue to finding meaning in suffering is the belief that suffering itself serves good ends. The reason for it does not depend on what caused it but what it produces. "That which doesn't kill me makes me better" is one expression of this attitude. The ordeals of suffering can purify us, make us reach heights and depths otherwise unknowable. It makes us grow. It develops our souls. It is "humanizing." (Perhaps *The Death of Ivan* Ilych [Tolstoy, 1886/1971] can be read as an account of what the human spirit can gain by going through the suffering brought about by the imminence of death.) For Christians, the suffering of Christ brought about the salvation of all his people: His passion, reenacted each year in the rituals surrounding Easter, had profound meaning because He suffered and died for mankind. Similarly, a belief in Reincarnation sees the life I am living now as preparation for my next life. What I suffer in this life will send me into the next one on a higher level. Likewise, all self-sacrifice is based on the belief that I choose my suffering in order to achieve some worthy end.

These are some—though far from all—of the themes to be encountered, explored, expressed in literary works. The question is why a person preparing to be a caregiver needs the kinds of understanding—the intuitions and insights—to be acquired by participating thus vicariously in other lives than his or her own. The simple answer seems to be that after such extended experience, the caregiver will have an extended capacity to relate to other human beings with the qualities we consider essentially human.

William Faulkner, accepting the Nobel Prize for Literature in 1950, talks about these qualities, a major subject in all his works, and about the special function of literature in disseminating "old universal truths." He calls upon young writers "already dedicated to the . . . anguish and travail" involved in writing to consider it their duty "to write about these things," to communicate them to their readers, to "help man endure by lifting his heart, by reminding him of the courage and honor and hope and pride and compassion and pity and sacrifice which have been the glory of his past" (p. 195)—all truths of which human beings should be constantly mindful.

The practical question remains: What difference will this kind of knowledge and understanding make in your care of your patients? This question, in all honesty, is impossible to answer. "Felt understanding" is qualitatively different from knowledge leading to skills in medical procedures whose benefits are immediate and clear. But, however subtly, such understanding undoubtedly will affect the attitudes you bring to your practice. You will know that no two patients in exactly the same situation share exactly the same background and outlook. You will respect the fact that you have no way of knowing what is going on in your patient's head unless he lets you know through words or behavior, both of which you may learn to interpret through your vicarious knowledge. You will certainly not try to counsel your patient to think or behave in some fashion agreeable to you, on some assumption that you share the same ways of regarding and interpreting experience.

Above all, your enlarged thinking, beliefs, attitudes will directly affect your attitudes and actions toward your patients and will effect an unspoken bond with them without need of words. Even the most well-intentioned words, in fact, may set up barriers between caregiver and patient. "I know how you feel," for example, falls all too glibly from the lips of sympathetic attendants speaking from their own experience only. A patient may doubt this easy statement and respond with withdrawal or even overt rejection: "You have no idea how I feel." This well-meaning person may well have unwittingly heightened the suffering by seeming to trivialize it.

One of our greatest American poets, Walt Whitman, has addressed this very question of the relationship between caregiver and patient/sufferer in his poem called "The Wound-Dresser" (1993). In real life, Whitman was himself a wound-dresser, a nurse, during the bloody events of the Civil War. This poem presents him, now an old man, trying to explain to young people what the experience was like. As we accompany him on his rounds through blood-soaked battlefields and through hospital tents and makeshift buildings, we come to realize that he is doing far more than tending wounds. What is it—a touch, a gesture, a glance, a word—that establishes such communion between him and those he attends? We sense that, in addition to alleviating pain, he somehow also eases the suffering of young men far from home and facing death, abandoned, isolated, hopeless. Is it that they feel he truly understands what they are going through, that he shares their humanity? Something there is that results in "many a soldier's loving arms about this neck" and "many a soldier's kiss . . . on these bearded lips" (p. 389).

Most likely, what is being demonstrated here is the consolation drawn from the shared humanity of sufferer and caregiver, this "wound-dresser" whose ability to identify with each sufferer establishes a communion that says, "Here is somebody who understands and cares." Such a person provides some haven when the top of one's world has blown off. It is this sense of shared humanity— we are all in this boat together—that gives final meaning to the term "care"giver and separates him/her from the rest of human kind, most of whom neither know of the suffering going on nor would truly care about it if they did.

W. H. Auden's poem, "Musee des Beaux Arts" (1945), gives poignant expression to this fact of life. Looking around at the "Old Masters" represented on the museum's walls, the poet observes "how well they understood [suffering's] human position" (p. 3). The rest of humanity are too much involved in living their own lives to care about or even notice suffering taking place right under their noses. The forsaken cry of Icarus, the boy with wings of wax who drops out of the sky after flying too close to the sun, falls on deaf ears: "It was not an important failure" for other people who themselves "had somewhere to get to" and would uncaringly move on.

Auden passes no judgment on this indifference. He simply describes the way things are, a fact of life. His poem, however, points to an essential difference between those going into some medical profession and the general populace. By choosing one of these professions, you commit yourself to care about the suffering of others.

Selected Poems

THE END OF THE WORLD
ARCHIBALD MACLEISH

Quite unexpectedly as Vasserot
The armless ambidextrian was lighting
A match between his great and second toe
And Ralph the lion was engaged in biting
The neck of Madame Sossman while the drum
Pointed, and Teeny was about to cough
In waltz-time swinging Jocko by the thumb—
Quite unexpectedly the top blew off.

And there, there overhead, there, there, hung over
Those thousands of white faces, those dazed eyes
There in the starless dark the poise, the hover,
There with vast wings across the canceled skies,
There in the sudden blackness the black pall
Of nothing, nothing, nothing—nothing at all (1952, p. 23).

THE LEG
KARL SHAPIRO

Among the iodoform, in twilight-sleep,
What have I lost? He first inquires,
Peers in the middle distance where a pain,
Ghost of a nurse hastily moves, and day,
Her blinding presence pressing in his eyes
And now his ears. They are handling him
With rubber hands. He wants to get up.

One day beside some flowers near his nose
He will be thinking, When will I look at it?
And pain, still in the middle distance, will reply,

At what? *And he will know it's gone,*
O where! And begin to tremble and cry.
He will begin to cry as a child cries
Whose puppy is mangled under a screaming wheel.

Later, as if deliberately, his fingers
Begin to explore the stump. He learns a shape
That is comfortable and tucked in like a sock.
This has a sense of humor, this can despise
The finest surgical limb, the dignity of limping,
The nonsense of wheel-chairs. Now he smiles to the wall;
The amputation becomes an acquisition.

For the leg is wondering where he is (all is not lost)
And surely he has a duty to the leg;
He is its injury, the leg is his orphan,
He must cultivate the mind of the leg,
Pray for the part that is missing, pray for peace
In the image of man, pray, pray for its safety,
And after a little it will die quietly.

The body, what is it, Father, but a sign
To love the force that grows us, to give back
What in thy palm is senselessness and mud?
Knead, knead the substance of our understanding
Which must be beautiful in flesh to walk
That if Thou take me angrily in hand
And hurl me to the shark, I shall not die! (1968, p. 82)

HAP

Thomas Hardy

If but some vengeful god would call to me
From up the sky, and laugh: "Thou suffering thing,
Know that thy sorrow is my ecstacy,
That thy love's loss is my hate's profiting!"
Then would I bear it, clench myself, and die,
Steeled by the sense of ire unmerited;
Half-eased in that a Powerfuller than I
Had willed and meted me the tears I shed.

But not so. How arrives it joy lies slain,
And why unblooms the best hope ever sown?
—Crass Casualty obstructs the sun and rain.
And dicing Time for gladness casts a moan . . ..
These purblind Doomsters had as readily strown
Blisses about my pilgrimage as pain (1976, p. 9).

THE WOUND-DRESSER
WALT WHITMAN

1

An old man bending I come among new faces,
Years looking backward resuming in answer to children,
Come tell us old man, as from young men and maidens that love me;
("Arous'd and angry, I'd thought to beat the alarum, and urge relentless war,
But soon my fingers fail'd me, my face droop'd, and I resign'd myself,
To sit by the wounded and sooth them, or silently watch the dead;)
Years hence of these scenes, of these furious passions, these chances,
Of unsurpass'd heroes, (was one side so brave? The other was equally brave;)
Now be witness again, paint the mightiest armies of earth,
Of those armies so rapid so wondrous what saw you to tell us?
What stays with you latest and deepest? Of curious panics
Of hard-fought engagements or sieges tremendous what deepest remains?

2

O maidens and young men I love and that love me,
What you ask of my days those the strangest and sudden your talking recalls,
Soldier alert I arrive after a long march cover'd with sweat and dust,
In the nick of time I come, plunge in the fight, loudly shout in the rush of successful charge,

Enter the captur'd works—yet lo, like a swift-running river they fade,
Pass and are gone they fade—I dwell not on soldiers' perils or soldiers' joys,
(Both I remember well—many the hardships, few the joys, yet I was content.)

But in silence, in dreams' projections,
While the world of gain and appearance and mirth goes on,
So soon what is over forgotten, and waves wash the imprints off the sand,
With hinged knees returning I enter the doors, (while for you up there,
Whoever you are, follow without noise and be of strong heart).

Bearing the bandages, water and sponge,
Straight and swift to my wounded I go,
Where they lie on the ground after the battle brought in,
Where their priceless blood reddens the grass the ground,
Or to the rows of hospital tent, or under the roof'd hospital,
To the long rows of cots up and down each side I return,
To each and all one after another I draw near, not one do I miss,
An attendant follows holding a tray, he carries a refuse pail,
Soon to be filled with clotted rags and blood, emptied and fill'd again.

I onward go, I stop,
With hinged knees and steady hand to dress wounds,
I am firm with each, the pangs are sharp yet unavoidable,

One turns to me his appealing eyes—poor boy! I never knew you,
Yet I think I could not refuse this moment to die for you, if that would save
you.

3
On, on I go (open doors of time! open hospital doors!)
The crush'd head I dress, (poor crazed hand tear not the bandage away,)
The neck of the cavalry-man with the bullet through and through I examine,
Hard the breathing rattles, quite glazed already the eye, yet life struggles
hard,
(Come sweet death! be persuaded O beautiful death!
In mercy come quickly.)

From the stump of the arm, the amputated hand,
I undo the clotted lint, remove the slough, wash off the matter and blood,
Back on his pillow the soldier bends with curv'd neck and side-falling head,
His eyes are closed, his face is pale, he dares not look on the bloody stump,
And has not yet look'd at it.

I dress a wound in the side, deep, deep,
But a day or two more, for see the frame all wasted and sinking,
And the yellow-blue countenance see.

I dress the perforated shoulder, the foot with the bullet-wound,
Cleanse the one with a gnawing and putrid gangrene, so sickening, so
offensive,
While the attendant stands behind aside me holding the tray and pail.

I am faithful, I do not give out,
The fractur'd thigh, the knee, the wound in the abdomen,
These and more I dress with impassive hand, (yet deep in my breast a fire,
a burning flame.)

4
Thus in silence in dreams' projections,
Returning, resuming, I thread my way through the hospitals,
The hurt and the wounded I pacify with soothing hand,
I sit by the restless all the dark night, some are so young,
Some suffer so much, I recall the experience sweet and sad,
(Many a soldier's loving arms about this neck have cross'd and rested,
Many a soldier's kiss dwells on these bearded lips.) (1993, pp. 385–89)

MUSEE DES BEAUX ARTS
W. H. AUDEN

About suffering they were never wrong,
The Old Masters: how well they understood
Its human position; how it takes place
While someone else is eating or opening a window or just walking dully
along;

> *How, when the aged are reverently, passionately waiting*
> *For the miraculous birth, there always must be*
> *Children who did not specially want it to happen, skating*
> *On a pond at the edge of the wood;*
> *They never forgot*
> *That even the dreadful martyrdom must run its course*
> *Anyhow in a corner, some untidy spot*
> *Where the dogs go on with their doggy life and the torturer's horse*
> *Scratches its innocent behind on a tree.*
>
> *In Brueghel's Icarus, for instance: how everything turns away*
> *Quite leisurely from the disaster; the ploughman may*
> *Have heard the splash, the forsaken cry,*
> *But for him it was not an important failure; the sun shone*
> *As it had to on the white legs disappearing into the green*
> *Water; and the expensive delicate ship that must have seen*
> *Something amazing, a boy falling out of the sky,*
> *Had somewhere to get to and sailed calmly on (1943, p. 3).*

REFERENCES

Auden, W.H. (1945). Musee des Beaux Arts. In *The collected poetry of W.H. Auden.* (p. 3). New York: Random House.

Beckett, S. (1954). *Waiting for Godot.* New York: Grove Press.

The Holy Bible: King James version (1993). New York: American Bible Society.

Camus, A. (1991). The Myth of Sisyphus. In J. O'Brien. (trans.) *The Myth of Sisyphus and other essays.* (pp. 119–23). New York: Vintage Books.

Faulkner, W. (1960). The writer's duty. Nobel Prize acceptance speech, Stockholm, December 10, 1950. In W. Blair & J. Gerber. (Eds.). *Repertory.* (p. ix). Chicago: Random House.

Hardy, T. (1976). Hap. In J. Gibson. (Ed.). *The complete poems of Thomas Hardy.* (p. 9). New York: Macmillan Publishing Company.

MacLeish, A. (1952). The end of the world, from Streets of the moon. (1926). In *Collected poems, Boston.* (p. 23). Boston: Houghton-Mifflin, The Riverside Press.

MacLeish, A. (1956). *J.B..* Boston: Houghton-Mifflin, The Riverside Press.

Pope, A. (1711/1951). An essay on criticism. In L. Kroenberger (Ed.). *Alexander Pope: Selected works. Modern Library Edition.* (pp. 32–53). New York: Random House.

Shapiro, K. (1968). The leg. In *Collected poems, 1940–1978.* (p. 82). New York: Random House.

Tolstoy, L. (1886/1971). The death of Ivan Ilych. In L. Maude & A. Maude (trans.). *The death of Ivan Ilych and other stories.* (pp. 1–73). New York: Oxford University Press.

Whitman, W. (1993). The wound-dresser. In *Leaves of grass: The "deathbed" edition.* (pp. 385–89). New York: Random House, Modern Library.

OTHER RECOMMENDED READINGS

Lowry, M. (2000). *Under the volcano.* New York: Harper-Collins, Perennial Classics Series.

Under the Volcano is widely considered to be one of the greatest novels of the 20th century. Although not easy to read (much of it weaves in and out of its protagonist's mind in a fashion of writing called *stream-of consciousness*), it is well worth the trouble. Its remarkable rendition of the suffering of Geoffrey Firmin, "the Consul," enlarges into a picture of the 20th century itself. In the introduction, the English poet, Stephen Spender says of it:

> By the time we have finished this novel we know how a drunk thinks and feels, walks and lies down, and we experience not only the befuddledness of drinking but also its moments of translucent clairvoyance, perfected expression . . .. Fundamentally, *Under the Volcano* is no more *about* drinking than *King Lear* is *about* senility. It is about the Consul, which is another matter, for what we feel about him is that he is great and shattered. We also feel that he could have written the novel which describes his downfall, and this means that, considered as an art of consciousness attained, this is no downfall, but his triumph (p. ix).

As a matter of fact, we can say that the Consul did write the novel, for he is a thinly disguised version of Malcolm Lowry himself, whose suffering—far from making him better—eventually destroyed him because he would not or could not take the actions that would have saved him.

Pinter, H. (1968). *The caretaker.* London: Methuen.

Weales, G. (Ed.) 1967). *Arthur Miller: Death of a salesman; text and criticism.* New York: Harper-Collins, Perennial Classics Series.

BOOKS ABOUT INDIVIDUAL SUFFERING IN ILLNESS

Casey, J. (1982). *From why to yes.* New York: University Press of America.

Frank, A. (1991). *At the will of the body: Reflections on illness.* Boston: Houghton-Mifflin.

Gee, E. (1992). *Light around the dark.* New York: NLN.

Jaffe, H. (1994). *Why me? Why anyone?* Northvale, NJ: Jason Anderson.

Willig, J. (2001). *Lessons from the school of suffering.* Cincinnati: St. Anthony Messenger Press.

Index

Page numbers followed by an "f" indicate figures.